**DOCTOR
A. T. STILL
IN THE LIVING**

*Osteopathy is divine geometry, physics & chemistry*

*Robert E. Truhlar*

# *DOCTOR A. T. STILL IN THE LIVING*

## *HIS CONCEPTS AND PRINCIPLES OF HEALTH AND DISEASE*

*—An Annotated Version—*

COMPILED, EDITED, AND WITH AN INTRODUCTION BY

**Robert E. Truhlar, D. O.**

**All Worlds Press, LLC**
**Roswell, Georgia, USA**

Original Copyright © 1950
by Robert E. Truhlar

# all w●rlds
# -PRESS-

Annotated Version Published By
All Worlds Press LLC
Roswell, GA

The book *Doctor A. T. Still in the Living* is a public domain work.

The annotations and additions to this book *Doctor A. T. Still in the Living: An Annotated Version* are copyrighted.

Annotated Version Copyright © 2025 by All Worlds Press, LLC.
All rights reserved.

Book design by FreeAgentPress.com

ISBN: 978-1-963899-12-2

LCCN applied for

**Disclaimer**

The information in this book is for informational purposes only. The information in this book is not intended as a substitute for the advice provided by your physician or other healthcare professional. You should not use the information in this book for diagnosing or treating a health problem, mental-health issue, or disease; or for prescribing any medication or other treatment. The information in this book are the sole opinions of the authors and are not meant to represent the opinions or statements set forth by other individuals or organizations. Buying, reading, or listening to this book does not form a physician-patient relationship with Dr. Arlene Dijamco or Dr. James E. Gaydos. Consult with a healthcare professional directly before implementing any changes to your health regimen, and do not delay seeking treatment because of something you have read in this book. Neither the authors or the publisher shall be liable or responsible for any loss or damage allegedly arising from any information or suggestions in this book.

# Dedication

---

*This book is dedicated to*

*A.T. Still, the founder of osteopathy*

*Robert E. Truhlar, DO,
who compiled the original book*

*The many osteopaths that came before us*

*Our present teachers and colleagues*

*Our patients*

*And the future of osteopathy*

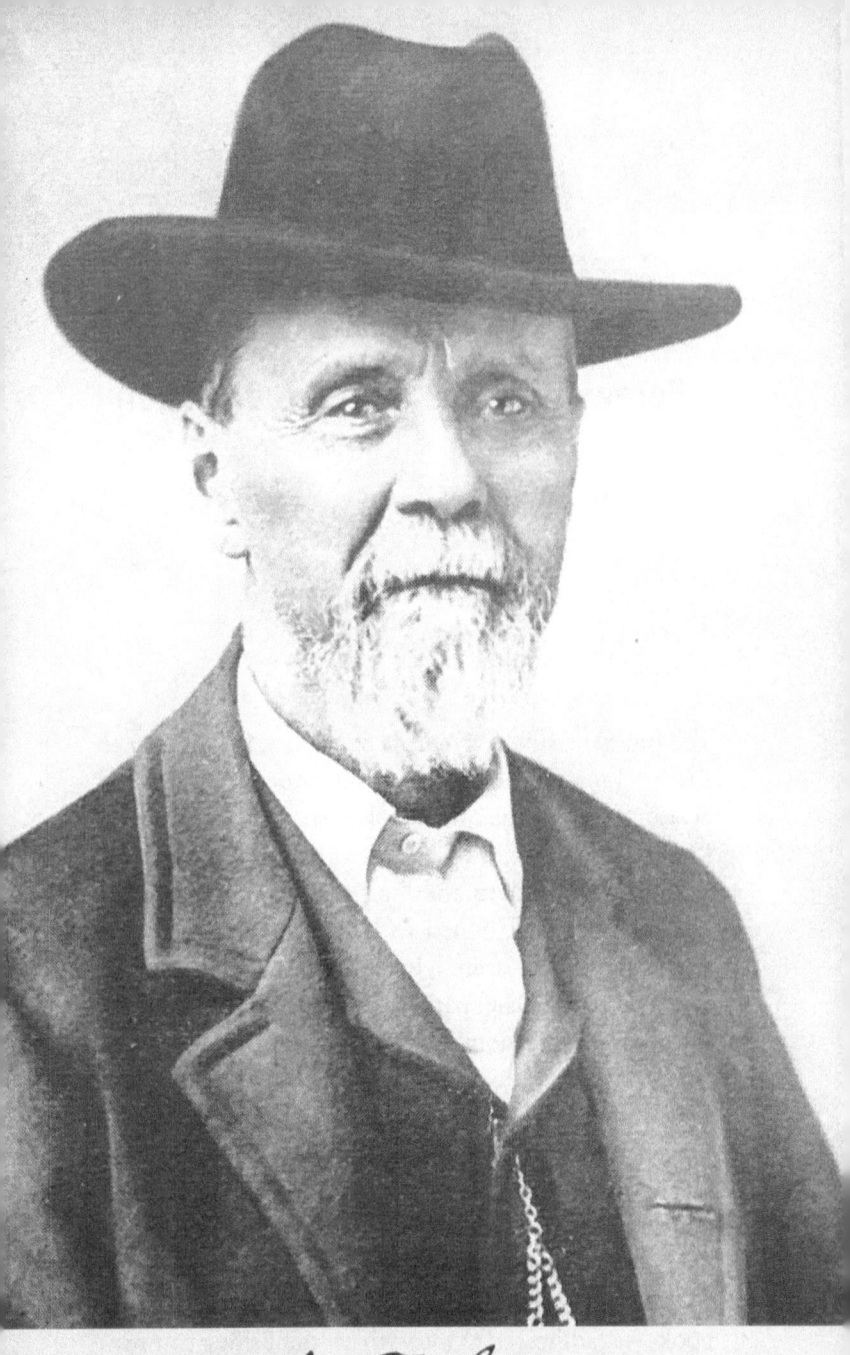

*A. T. Still.*
FOUNDER OF OSTEOPATHY

# Foreword to the Annotated Version

## By Arlene Dijamco, M.D.

The moment I held a reprint of *Doctor A. T. Still in the Living*, I read Dr. Truhlar's introduction and said aloud, "I want to re-publish this book with All Worlds Press." I felt that I was holding an Osteopathic gem. Here was a book dedicated to the "spiritual understanding" of Osteopathy, and I hoped to honor the work in a way that reflected its sacredness. "This book needs to be available to all Osteopaths," I said. I could already see the annotated version in my imagination.

The next few moments unfolded so quickly. First, I looked at the two packages in my hand. Strangely, I had received two copies in the mail. Hmmm… maybe I forgot and ordered it twice. I check my order history and no. I asked to see if a friend had sent me a copy. Also, no. Second, and even more intriguing was that one of the books was addressed to me with my publishing company name: All Worlds Press LLC. How was that possible?

All Worlds Press had never been added to my online address book. Was this a divine message or an unexplained glitch? It's all a matter of perspective, and for me it was a small miracle and nudge of encouragement.

As philosopher-physicians, we are each responding to a call from the Stillness—The Great I AM—in service to humanity. It is with deep gratitude that we walk on the path paved by Dr. Still and many others before us, as it takes courage to answer this calling. However, in doing so we feel alive! After all, to be an Osteopath does start with Be-ing. So, let us continue onward in our art.

I hope that the love and wisdom in this book will inspire us all to explore consciousness through Osteopathy, so that we may all be more pure expressions of our true essence. We are the Living Osteopathy.

In Stillness,

Arlene Dijamco, M.D.

# Foreword to the Annotated Version

## By James E. Gaydos, D.O.

I have always been fond of collecting aphorisms from Dr. Still, reciting them in a quiet moment during a hike, or reading indoors during inclement weather. In studying the thoughts that Dr. Still expressed, I discovered a self-renewal that I had not felt for years. Later, I enjoyed bringing some of these writings to workshops, and reading one aloud at the start of a meeting, or integrating another into a presentation. In time, Dr. Still's words became the common method to ground the class, and set a positive tone at the opening of an event.

Recently, I found a copy of Dr. Truhlar's book. His inscription is included in this copy. Just holding this book provided a powerful sense of Dr. Still's presence within its pages. From that time, discussions ensued on how to share these stories with the broader osteopathic community of dedicated colleagues, teachers, and students, and thus, the beginnings of this annotated book. Hopefully, meditating on Dr. Still's reflections and wise words will provide the same sense of grounding and self-renewal as we had appreciated in our smaller gatherings.

It is my heart-felt wish that you may experience deep inspiration from *Dr. A. T. Still in the Living*, and find our annotations meaningful in expanding and enriching your life and practice. This is Living Osteopathy where "Suns appear where you never saw a Star, brilliant in the Rays of God's Wisdom, as reflected in man and the laws of life…"

With Love,

James E. Gaydos, D.O.

# Suggestions for How to Use This Book

- This is a book of osteopathic meditations, as Dr. Robert E. Truhlar had envisioned.

- This is a book of osteopathic meditations, as Dr. Robert E. Truhlar had envisioned.

- Dr. Truhlar originally arranged this collection alphabetically based upon key words which we have **bolded** throughout the book. We also realized that it might be practical to be able to search for these individual bolded terms, so we created an index for that purpose. Consider perusing this book in various ways whether by reading line by line, searching terms in the index, browsing the annotations, or opening to a random page. These are meant to help make Dr. Still's living words even more accessible to you.

- At times, Dr. A.T. Still used "God" to refer to "Spirit." This book is not meant to support any particular religious orientation, it simply acknowledges that we are all spiritual beings. Our intentions are for readers from all backgrounds to be able to enjoy this book.

- Note that some of the language used in Dr. Still's time might differ from our usage today. For excerpts that might seem puzzling, confusing, curious, or particularly intriguing, we have included expanded references in the annotations section. These references are meant to give further context to the passages in this book.

- We realize that some readers may want to record and collect their own annotations. In that light, there are additional spaces in the margins to add your own impressions.

- This book is meant to help us Dig On and Dream On, inspired by the wisdom, ideals, concepts, and dreams of Dr. Still: keeping the Stillness alive within us, in our practices, and in our everyday lives. This is the Living Osteopathy.

# Preface

## By Robert E. Truhlar, D.O.

The compilation of this volume was prompted by talks, over breakfast and luncheon tables at our conventions. Many of the older Doctors expressed the feeling that there must be a greater "spiritual understanding" of Osteopathy in the profession.

Dr. Andrew Taylor Still had this understanding of the human body as created by the "Divine Architect", many of the older men and the successful ones in our profession have this "spiritual concept."

In studying and meditating upon these aphorisms, maxims, parables and similitudes, submerge your materialistic and fundamentalistic consciousness, walk hand in hand with Dr. Still, as he walked with God, that you too may walk in the light of understanding and reason as he did.

This volume in a small measure will show the deep understanding and wisdom that Dr. Still had of disease. It is for posterity to review, consider, evaluate and meditate upon, for the development and improvement in the art of healing.

These capsules of wisdom and knowledge must be preserved for those who come after us, they are the guideposts of the Osteopathic way of life, just as they have been for us and others before us.

A natural law is omniscient always, knowing the cause and what to do.

A natural law is omnipresent with and works by the media involved in its sphere of operations.

A natural law is omnipotent of a force always present within and without that is absolute concerning the organism or purpose it represents.

We have the degree D.O. following our names of signatures, it means more than Doctor of Osteopathy and I feel that it meant something else to Dr. Still.

Demonstrating Omniscience.

Demonstrating Omnipresence.

Demonstrating Omnipotence.

These are the real meaning of D.O. as demonstrated and taught by our beloved founder Dr. Andrew Taylor Still.

Those that have eyes let them see; those that have ears let them hear.

ROBERT E. TRUHLAR, D.O.

*"In seventy-five years in the crucible of time, not one statement made by Dr. A. T. Still has needed revising."*

**—WILLIAM G. SUTHERLAND, D.O.**

# Acknowledgment

We wish to express our sincere thanks and appreciation to the Doctors in the field, who responded to the call for material, to make this volume possible.

# A

"An osteopath reasons from his knowledge of **anatomy**."

"The rule of the **artery** must be absolute, universal, and unobstructed, or disease will be the result."

"There is not a known **atom** in the whole human make-up that has not been propelled by the heart through the channels provided for such purposes."

"Ammonia an **antidote** for rattle-snake poison. Sulphuric-acid with three parts water kills the virus. Also good in rabies."

"Before you can go out into the world and fight the fight, you must master human **anatomy** and physical laws."

"The Grand **Architect** of the Universe builds without sound of hammer; nature is silent in her work."

"Give me the **age** of God and I will give you the **age** of Osteopathy."

"The highest officer in command is the **artery** of nourishment, which must be **assisted** by the nerve of motion and the vein of renovation."

"A disturbed **artery** marks the beginning to an hour and a minute when disease began to sow its seeds of destruction in the human body."

"The **artery** is the father of the rivers of life, health and ease, and its impure or muddy water is first in all disease."

"Osteopathy is king of **asthma**."

"The **arteries** bring the blood and wash it with the spirit of life."

"It is the ignorance of and the inattention to the **arteries** to supply and the veins to carry away deposits that lead to the formation of tumors in the lungs, abdomen, or any part of the system."

"Is not the labor of the **artery** complete when it has fed the hungry nerves? The nerves gestate and send forth all substances that are applied by Nature in the construction of man."

"Of what use is a knowledge of **anatomy** to a man if he overlooks cause and effect in the results obtained by the body machinery."

"The only **assistance** others can give you, will be a better understanding of the fundamental principles upon which Osteopathy is founded."

"A knowledge of **anatomy** with its applications covers every inch of ground that is necessary to qualify you to become a skillful and successful Osteopath, when you go forth into the world to combat diseases."

"If the carotid **artery** should tire out and not be able to perform its duty the brain would tire out also, and cease to operate."

"You will find making the bony **adjustment** to be the easiest part about Osteopathy. All you have to do is to carry them through their normal physiological range of motion without force or injury, keeping in mind any joint carried much less forced beyond its normal range of motion. The ligaments are injured beyond repair."

"An Osteopathic **adjustment** is and must be one of precision."

"My highest **ambition** is heaven and an **automobile**."

"The Osteopathic physician removes the obstruction and lets Nature's remedy — **Arterial** blood — be the doctor."

"The **Anatomy** text (Gray) you are studying is one of the Standard Anatomies of the world and it states that the sacro-iliac joint is an immovable joint and I stand here alone and expect you to support me that the sacro-iliac joint is a moveable joint and that all the **Anatomies** will be changed before many years, stating that it is a movable joint and is the cause of sciatica in many cases. I may not live to see it but some of you will." (His prediction came true as all the standard anatomies include it today.)

"**Adjuncts** are not necessary to the Osteopath."

"The importance of injuries to the hip are too much overlooked. To the Osteopath it should be a subject of the deepest thought." [**anatomy**]

"First loosen the dislocated end from other tissues; then gently bring it back to its original place." [**anatomy**]

"My **advice** is to let your object be to keep out of papers and do good work today and better work tomorrow and your patients will multiply just in proportion to your ability to demonstrate that you know your business."[1]

"I want to emphasize to you each and all that if you pull and haul your **asthmatic** patients everyday, you will surely fail."

"Spend fifteen minutes to one half hour in palpitation of the spine." [**anatomy**]

"Don't **ape** others. Fit yourself to do what others cannot do."

A knowledge of **anatomy** is all you want or need, as it is all you can use or ever will use in your practice although you may live one hundred years."

"Oh! Lord give me more **anatomy** each day I live, because experience has taught me the unavoidable demands when in the 'sick room'."

"Begin with the **atlas**, follow with the search-light of quickened reason, comb back your hair of mental strength, and never leave that bone till you have learned how many nerves pass thru and around that wisely formed first part of the neck. Remember it was planned and built by the mind and hand of the Infinite."

"If we understand **anatomy** as we should, we know man is the greatest engine ever produced, complete in form, an electro-magnet, a motor and would be incomplete if it could not burn its own gases."

"If an **artery** cannot unload its contents a strain follows, and as an artery must have room to deposit its supplies it proceeds to build other vessels adjacent to the points of obstruction."

"**Arterial** motion is normal during all **ages**, from the quick pulse of the baby's arm to the slow pulse of the aged."[2]

"The study of the framework of the chest should be done with the greatest care." (**anatomy**)

# B

"You cut your finger: Hello **blood**! Where did you come from? From that biscuit you ate this morn. Now tell me what process that biscuit went thru from the time you ate it, till blood showed up."

Some of the public had been concerned about him wearing **boots** and he said he never, "could see why the public should be concerned whether he wore one pant's leg inside his boot and the other outside, for they were his pants and he felt it was his privilege to wear them in any manner he pleased."

"And don't forget that God gave you **brains**."

"I dissected many **bodies** so as to better understand and often improve on the books I read."

"Boys, a little more **brain** and less **brawn**."

About the **brain** of a man who had been used to success in all things, "This is of no use to others, it is no better than others only in one way, he had the courage to use it and let all others alone."

"He who talks much and does little, and hates his successful **brother or sister**, because they have succeeded by perseverance while he has failed through stupidity, will never succeed in anything."

"Every **blood** vessel is accompanied and controlled by forces suited to the system of **blood** supply."

"Look upon the human body as an organized brotherhood of laborers. The **business** of the operator is to keep peace and harmony throughout the whole **brotherhood**."

"To know of a **bone** in its entirety would close both ends of an eternity."

"The **brain** of man was God's drugstore and had in it all liquids, drugs, lubricating oils, opiates, acids and anti-acids, and every quality of drugs that the wisdom of God thought necessary for human happiness and health."[3]

"I learned the lesson and it was the most valuable lesson in my life, that one's **brain** is his own reliance. It is a judge that will give a careful studied opinion to me."

"Of all parts of the **body** of man, the **brain** should be the most attractive. It is the place where all forces center, where all nerves are connected with one common battery."

"Examine and see if you don't find a **button** there that can govern cold and heat."

"The living **blood** swarmed with corpuscles to all parts of the **body**."

"**Blood** is an unknown red or black fuid, found inside of the human body, in tubes, channels, or tunnels. What it is, how it is made and what it does in the arteries after it leaves the heart, before it returns to the heart thru the veins, is one of the mysteries of animal life."

"Without knowing the functions of the **brain**, we cannot know its uses."

"The day thou eatest anything else, thou shalt surely die. Stick to the **brotherhood**."

"We must run with all the rivers of **blood** that travel thru the system."

"We must start our exploring **boat** with the **blood** of the aorta and float with this vital current, and watch the unloading of supplies, for the diaphragma and all that is under it."

"How is **blood** driven to the heart and returned to the place from whence it started?"

"One's **brain** is his only reliance."

"If you **burst** a **boiler** by high pressure or other-wise, your engine ceases to move. And just the same of an over-worked brain or body."

"We **believe** only when we do not know. **Belief** and doubt are equal terms."

"Let your search-light ever shine **bright** on the **brain**. On it we must depend for power."

"Unobstructed **blood** cannot form a tumor, nor allow inharmony to dwell in any part of the system."

"The first step in Osteopathy is a **belief** in our own **body**."[4]

"In quality and quantity, you may find the **blood stream** normal as revealed by the laboratory tests, but if it isn't moving on time, there is the beginning of disorder and disorder is the **beginning** of disease. For the rule of the artery is supreme."

"Snapping and popping of the **bones** is no evidence of an adjustment."

"Never mind what the book says, God gave you a **brain**."[5]

"Pure arterial **blood** is to me nothing more nor less than the living seeds of life, as much so as the seed of the mustard, wheat or any vegetable seed known to the agriculturist."

"I want to emphasize to the student or operator the absolute unqualified importance of knowing the duties and responsibilities of a **bone** in keeping up its part as a laboratory and **building**."

"One asks, 'How must we pull a **bone** to replace it'? I reply, 'Pull it to its proper place and leave it there'."

"That 'popping' is no criterion to go by. **Bones** do not always pop when they go back to their proper place nor does it mean they are properly adjusted when they do 'pop'."

"In adjusting **bones** the mechanic is governed by three principles—the lever, the screw, and the wedge."

"If you want to show your wife's **brains**—bring in her **babes**."

"Every atom of **blood** when sent forth from the lungs is a living seed, as much so as the seed of any shrub, flower or tree in all nature."

"Where do the atoms of **blood** receive that perfection which is the seedlike property of the atom by which when planted in proper soil it will vegetate, grow and produce what we call tissue, bone and muscle and all constructed substances?"

"Is a **bone** personally responsible in performing any duty **beyond** its service as a **brace** or support for the body while in the erect position? Does its personality extend beyond that purpose? Is it a house in which a process of manufacturing substances for repairing takes place? Does it construct its own habitation?"

"In order to have good arterial **blood** the lungs must receive good wholesome food from the abdomen."

"Let us reason that at conception every organ of the whole human **body** enters one great labor union. They labor and do faithful and good work until one member of the union is mistreated. Then the whole **brotherhood** comes to a halt to consult, and it never compromises, until the doctor sets all things right, or apologizes for his failures and calls counsel."

"Remember that during childbirth the **bladder** is often drawn down, and closes the water ducts from the kidneys to the bladder, and it is our work to put all these soft parts in place."[6]

"Consult the nerve and **blood** supply to and from the brain and govern yourself accordingly."

"We must arrange our **bodies** in such true lines that ample Nature can select and associate, by its definite measures and weights and its keen powers of choice and kinds, that which can make all the fluids needed for our bodily uses, from the crude **blood** to the active flame of life, as they are seen when marshalled for duty, obeying the edicts of the mind of the Infinite."

"With all the combined intelligence of man, we cannot make one drop of **blood**, because we do not know what it is."

"We can analyze material **bodies** but we have to stop at the life line for more knowledge."

"Of all officers of life, none have greater duties to perform than the quarter-master of **blood** supply, who **borrows** the force with which he runs his deliveries from the brain which gives motion to all parts of active life."

"We are told by chemistry that two gases make water for the uses of the **body**."

"The **brain** flushes the nerves of the lymphatics first, and more than other system of the body."[7]

"No **blood** can pass thru a vein that is closed by resistance. Nor can it ever do it until resistance is suspended."

"The **body** generates its own heat and modulates to sweet climate and season."

"Has not your acquaintance with the human **body** opened your mind's eye to observe that in the laboratory of the human **body**, the most wonderful chemical results are being accomplished every day, minute and hour of your life?"

To think implies action of the **brain**. We can grade thought, altho we cannot measure its speed."

"Slaves and savages seldom fall victims to paralysis of any kind, but escape, for they know nothing of the strain of mind and hurried nutrition."[8]

"We must pass thru the waters of the Dead Sea by way of the Vena Cava, and observe the **boats** loaded with exhausted and worn-out blood, as it is passed in and channeled back to the heart."

"The organized substances in the human **body**, to the student of Osteopathy, should be in divisions when he **begins** to philosophize as an operator."

"**Building** and healthy renovation are united in a perpetual effort to construct and sustain purity. In these two are the facts and truths of life and health."

# C

"If I should give **calomel**, I would do it with my eyes shut and I would want to keep them shut for nine days, so uncertain would I be as to results. If you consider me a mesmerist, a big dose of pills may carry the thought away."[9]

"Every drug tolerated by an Osteopath in a disease will shake the **confidence** of your most intelligent patients, and always cause them to take your words, skill and ability at a great discount."

"**Cancer** begins long before recognized symptoms can be detected. When positively diagnosed, it may have spread its seeds in other parts of the body like a brush pile on fire. It will burst forth its sparks to other areas producing more fire. Cancer is first a local disease when it can be cured by surgery. When it becomes general, it is beyond human efforts. Cancer like other diseases does not develop in a normal tissue environment. There must be a stasis of lymphatic and venous flow. Treat all new growths with respect. Eliminate them with good surgery and careful dissection and procure normalcy of the human body."

"When a **cat** gets his tail caught in a door, don't say, 'poor kitty', or try to appease its pain by petting it. Open the door and turn it loose. You are Osteopaths, and thus get at the cause."

"A pain in the head is an effect. **Cause** is older than effect, and is absolute in all varations (sic) from the normal conditions."

"I wouldn't take one thousand dollars for the caw, caw of **crows** that have croaked at me; they simply act as manure to enrich my life-work."

"You should know the **cause** of a disease and be able to remove it."

"All **channels** to and from the heart must be cleared from all hindrances."

"Has **chemistry** ever detected a failure in the normal process in preparing the fluids of life? Has it ever found imperfection in the fluid itself or any part or principle of the whole economy of life?"

"Every **corpuscle** goes like a man in the army, with full instructions where to go, and with unerring precision it does its work, whether it be in the formation of a hair or the throwing of a spot of delicate tinting at certain distances on a peacocks back."

"He (God) simply endows the **corpuscles** with mind, and in obedience to His law each one of these soldiers of life goes to the duty he is to perform. It travels its beaten line without interfering with the work of others."

"Any variation from health has a cause and the **cause** has a location. It is the business of the Osteopath to locate and remove it (cause), doing away with the disease and getting health instead."

"The one who would deal in **conjectures** should be placed in the proper category to which he belongs, which is the driftwood that floats down the dark river overshadowed by the nightmare of doubt and superstition."

"I would advise you to bathe your heads long and often in the rivers of divine **confidence** and pray God to take care of you with other weak-minded people, who pretend to know that which they have not studied."

"Did you ever see a **coon** climb two trees at one time?"

"**Courage** is the gem that will set off your bosom."

"If in the human body you can find the most wonderful **chemical** laboratory that mind can conceive, why not give more of your time to that subject in order that you may have a better understanding of its workings?"

"I begin at the little toe with the view of giving you a homeopathic dose on obstructed **circulation** as evidence of the cause of heart disturbance."

"A tumefying **condition** undoubtedly marks the beginning of all catarrhal conditions."

"To **construct** wisely is natural to all beings."

"We will save time and grow wiser in **comprehension** and good results by cutting hay in the summer and killing hogs in the winter."

"I think that the cause of **croup** is largely the result of abnormality of the **cerumen** system."[10]

"My aim is to carefully explore all and never leave until I find the **cause** and use that which Nature's hand has placed on its workings and never overlooking small packages, as they often contain precious gems."

"Do **contagions** or contagious diseases come from seeds of matter or from changes of the powers of life, life-activities being modified by force of compounds that have been driven from natural channels, and creating new or abnormal activities that unite substances into other compounds that are poisonous?"

"We have reason to believe that all **contagious** diseases seek the lungs to pasture and deposit their germs. With the knowledge of how and where the germ is deposited, how it is fed and grows to universal occupancy of the system, we have but little to seek, except to know how to work the machinery and cause it to unload."

"Do not tell me you cannot put your fingers upon the **cause**."

"I contend that the **curing** comes direct from the liberation of the interspinous and costal nerves freed from bone pressure on the nerves of motion, sensation and nutrition."

"**Cause** is older than effect and is absolute in all variations from normal **conditions**."

"He had a **constipation** of ideas and diarrhea of words."

"There were those who were like squirrels, 'trying to **climb** two trees at once', those who were getting lost in 'no man's land'."

"Lets [*sic*] keep our **colleges** so different that they will have no appeal to those who want M.D. degrees."

"I think it is high time that we take our eyes off the smoke and hunt until we find the fire that produces the effect." (**cause**)

"If all writers acknowledge they do not know the **cause** producing such disease, why not drop them out and use the compass of reaction to find the road that leads to the cause producing such effects?"

"More **cripples** are produced by the use of too thick a diaper than people who do not reason from effect to cause have any idea of."[11]

"We will stick to the belief that Nature's **chemistry** can produce and apply the substance that will destroy any germ that appears in the various kinds of disease on which it is claimed they are found."

"By **chemistry** we learn to comprehend some of the laws of union in Nature which we can use with confidence."

"In **chemistry** we become acquainted with the law of cause and change in union, which is a standard law sought by the students of Osteopathy."

"Osteopathy believes that all parts of the human body act on **chemical compounds**, and from the general supply manufactures the substances for local wants."

"I think **consumption** begins by closing the channels of the **cerebro-spinal fluid** in the neck, which fluid starts as one of, if not the most highly refined elements in animal bodies."[12]

"We adjust the machinery and depend upon Nature's **chemical** laboratory for all elements necessary to repair, give ease and comfort, while nature's corpuscles do all the work necessary."

"Not only can Nature's **chemistry** destroy the germs but it can disorganize and pass away unnatural accumulations of lime."

"When medical schools find a growth or ulcer, they hunt for knife and caustic, cut and burn. You see at once that the theory is to combat the effect, and not the **cause**."

"**Clairvoyance** is mental X-radiance."

"The body has its own **chemical** laboratory, and man cannot improve it."

# D

"I reasoned that all the **drugs** man needed were put in him by nature's quartermaster, and that the supply was abundant, but our knowledge was limited of how to use the remedy nature had provided for us."

"Early in life I began to hate drugs."W

"There is now no **drug**, nor never will be whereby any chemical can balance and correct structural abnormalities that affect functions adversely."

"When all parts of the human body are in line we have perfect health. When they are not, the effect is **disease**. When the parts are readjusted disease gives place to health."

"Watch the fourth **dorsal**."

"You do not need drugs. The blood has a hundred **drugs** of its own of which the doctor knows nothing. But the body's drugs actually cure disease, whereas the doctor's drugs kill."

"**Death** is the completed work of development of the sum total of effort to a finished work of nature."

"If the supply channels of the body be obstructed and the life-giving currents do not reach their **destination** full-freighted, then disease sets in."

"Man should study and use the drugs of his **drug** store only."

"All **diseases** are only effects."

"Interfere with the current of blood and you steam down the river of life and land in the ocean of **death**."

"God is no **drug** doctor."

"**Disease** is only too much dirt in the wheels of life."

"**Disease** is evidently sown as atoms of gas, fluids or solids."

"The cause of **disease** has been for all ages a silent mystery, lying in ambush and shooting its smokeless powder and with its deadly bullets slaying its countless millions."

"All **digestion** is the result of electric shocks, sent forth from the brain by way of the motor system of nerves."

"Previous to all **discoveries** there exists the demand for the discovery."

"What has the **diaphragm** to do with good or bad health? The diaphragm surely gives much food for one who would search for the great 'whys' of disease."

"All parts of the body have a direct or indirect connection with the **diaphragm**."

"Each engine has a sacred duty to perform, under the penal law of **death** to itself and all other divisions of the whole being, man."

"**Disease** is just as liable to begin its work in the fascia and epithelium as at any other place."

"The **diaphragm** says: 'By me you live and by me you die. I hold in my hands the power of life and death. Acquaint now thyself with me and be at ease'."

"If nature requires **drugs**, where would it go to find the laboratory that could be trusted to make drugs that would benefit the body?"

"If we find a failure in health, we would surely show wisdom by going into the machine-shop to find **defects** in the machine or system of organs which starts with the crude material and brings forth pure blood."

"Explosion and **death** take place when union with fluids of other cells of different kinds occur."

"The use of **drugs** is not a science, let us call it a 'trade'."

"Viewed through the most powerful microscope or otherwise, no defects can be found in the works of the **Deity**."

"To cure **disease**, the abnormal parts must be adjusted to the normal."

"We say **disease** when we should say effect; for disease is the effect of a change in the parts of the physical body."

"**Disease** in an abnormal body is just as natural as is health when all parts are in place."

"**Disease** is the result of anatomical abnormalities followed by physiological discord."

"A sore tongue, sore eyes, sore tonsils, sore nose, running ears, the nasal air passages, and all the membranes rapidly heal when you have secured perfect **drainage**."

"The **doctor** of Osteopathy may fail, but the science never. As thought is, so is the deed; as the thing made is good or bad, so is its maker."

"An Osteopath must find the true corners as set by the **Divine** Surveyor."

"When we use the word, **'disease'** we mean anything that makes an unnatural showing in the body by pain."

"We must ever remember the **demands** of nature on the lymphatics, liver and kidneys."

"The **difficult** part about Osteopathy is in acquiring the intimate knowledge and understanding of the structures and the fluid and forces that govern their action."

"You cannot have too much of **dissection**. It will help you to verify your mental conception of the body's structure. But I want you to remember that the structures have an entirely different appearance and feel in **death** than in life."

"To be able to intelligently prescribe any and all **drugs**, one must first learn the fundamental principles that govern their administration. Namely:

There must exist within the body the physiological wrong for which the drug is given. Otherwise, it becomes a poison instead of a remedial agency and that is a life-time job for any man or woman."

"The best **doctor** is one who can help Nature cure itself."

"Bacteria do not cause **disease** as they are the "Turkey Buzzards' of the body, and live on dead cells."[13]

"In all cases of **indigestion** you will find tenderness in the region of the solar plexus."

"When morphine enters the body it takes possession, and says to the blood in the venous system, 'Keep still', and to the cellular system and excretory ducts, 'Be quiet, and they are still as far as misery is concerned. But during quietness vegetable fermentation proceeds with its work, carries on **decomposition** and the congestion becomes general instead of local and death scores another victory."

"A filthy sewer will produce **disease** in the whole city, so the failure of one organ will produce disease of the whole body, and the salvation of the city or body, depends on your mechanical philosophy and work."

"What is **death** but a birth from the second placenta to which life has been attached."

"The symptomatologist comes forward and describes, classifies and names the **disease** and prescribes his remedies. We ask him why he did not give us those names a week sooner. His answer is, We have to wait long for the disease to develop before we are warranted in giving names."

"**Drunkenness** is no disgrace but it is proof that the man has a disease, and the failure in the free circulation of his blood has allowed his liver and spleen to retain chalk, lime and earthy substances, and has prevented the manufacturing of healthy fluids where work is to keep the chalk and lime in a fluid condition and pass them off through the excretory system."

"As Nature always presents itself to our minds as seeds deposited in soil and season to suit, and it is loyal to its own laws only, we are constrained by this method of reasoning to conclude that **disease** must have a soil in which to plant its seeds before gestation and development."

"The **diaphragm** is possibly the least understood as being the cause of more diseases, when its supports are not all in line and normal position, than any other part of the body."

"It is only in keeping with reason that without a healthy **diaphragm** both in its form and action, disease is bound to be the result."

"When it becomes necessary to break the friendly relationship between life and matter, nature closes up the channels of supply." [**digestion**]

"As it becomes necessary to throw off oppressive governments, it becomes just as necessary to throw off other useless practices and customs." [**digestion**]

"**Digestion** is food reduced to atoms of gas both by chemical union and animal heat. The stomach is a finely constructed gas-retort."

"When a child dies by **disease**, he dies all at once."

"Electric shocks in **digestion** are in perpetual motion from the center of the earth to the soul of the surface. Not only do these shocks tear asunder all substances found in the alimentary channel, but they impart, inject and associate a moving principle called vitality."[14]

"Nature has placed its manufactories above a given line in the breast, and **develops** the crude materials below that line."

# E

An osteopath is only a human **engineer**, who should understand all the laws governing his engine and thereby master disease."

"There is no part which if affected by disease does not present a philosophical question to be answered by an **engineer** and not by an imitator nor a masseur."

"We as **engineers**, have but one question to ask, 'What has the body failed to do'?"

"To comprehend this **engine** of life or man which is so constructed with all conveniences for which it was made, it is necessary to constantly keep the plan and specifications before the mind, and in the mind, to such a degree that there is no lack of knowledge of the bearings and uses of all parts."

"**Electricity** is the force that is naturally required to contract muscles and force gases from the body."

"Is action produced by **electricity** put in motion, or is it the active principle that comes as spiritual man?"

"For what purpose did God make **ear-wax**? Is it food or refuse? If food, what is nourished by it? And how do you know your position is true and undebatable?"[15]

"Life means **existence**. Existence means subsistence. Subsistence means something to subsist upon and of the degree of refinement to suit the skilled work which is found marked on the trestleboard of the wisest of builders, whose work is absolutely correct in form and action and beautiful to behold. It calls out the administration of man and God himself, who did say of man, 'Not only good, but very good."

"Is this substance which is commonly called **ear-wax** technically called cerumen, dead, or is it alive while in the visible form? If dead, why and how did it lose its life? When alive is it in the gaseous or fluid state? And when alive and consumed as nutriment by the system, what does it nourish?"

"Why is it deposited in the center of the brain, if not to impart its vital principle to all nerves interested in life and nutrition both physical and vital. Its location, in itself, would indicate its importance." (**ear-wax**)

"When we examine a person paralyzed on one side, why do we find this bread of life (**ear-wax**) in such great quantities and not consumed? Have not one half of the brain and nerves of that whole side, limbs and all, lost their power of digestion?"

"The uses and importance of healthy **ear-wax** as a cure for disease has not had the attention of any author or disease or physiology, so far as I can find."

"**Edema** is one word that appears at the first showing of life and death in animal forms."

"**Edema** surely begins with the first tardy atom of matter."

"The cerebro-spinal fluid is one of the highest known **elements** that are contained in the human body, and unless the brain furnishes this fluid in abundance, a disabled condition of the body will remain. He who is able to reason will see that this great river of life must be tapped and the withering field irrigated at once or the harvest of health be forever lost."

"No known **element** can cause the decay of rust."

"As an **electrician** controls electric currents, so an Osteopath controls life currents and revives suspended forces."

"Think of yourself as an **electric** battery."

"Let your eyes be a microscope of the highest known power."

"Man must use his head and legs if he wants to succeed in any **enterprise**."

"You may find much that has never been written or practised before, but all such discoveries are truths born with the birth of **eternity**, old as God, and as true as life."

"You are **engineers**, not engine wipers."

"The internal mammary feeds the **eye**."[16]

"I have long believed that an **engineer** of the human body was the sick man's only hope."

"When **ego** comes in, conceit usually follows forcing respect out."

"Let me **eat** quick and trot, and I will have health and strength."

"We can now talk around and all over the **earth** by the power of the dreaded thunder and lightning. By it we travel, by it we see at night, by it we search on land and sea for friend or foe; in fact, it is dreadful no more but sought, used and loved by all who know of its uses in civil life."

"With the best **eye** of reason we see but dimly into the breast of man which contains the heart, the wonder of man and the secret of life."

"Why singing and roaring of **ears** in heart diseases, if there is no waste of pectoral **electricity**?"

"Neither the circulatory nor the nervous system have a fixed stability; both have a very sensitive **equilibrium** of necessity, must be so, to meet the changing **environment** of life."

"Can you say that any part has no importance physiologically, in this the greatest **engine** ever produced—the engine of human life?"

"Why do one person's **eyes** when congested become abnormally large and a constant stream of tears pass from them? Where is the friction responsible for this unnatural appearance of the eye? Would you go to the nerve and blood supply of the eye for the cause or would you cut those eyes out and throw them away?"

"As nerve **energy** is the soul and body of all digestion as far as man knows, we will see the importance of keeping all parts of the frame, every joint, every muscle and all connecting ligaments in perfect position without a twist or strain."

"If you comprehend your business as an **engineer** you will spend no time analyzing the steam or tar and the worn-out grease that comes out of the axles or off the piston rods, to see what is the matter with the engine."

"The **engineer** has to control the **engine** that produces small-pox, chicken-pox, measles, mumps, whooping-cough, diphtheria, laryngitis, pharyngitis, tonsilitis, tumors of the nose, disease of the tongue, throat, mouth, eyes, and all of the organs of the face and head."

"I never found a bed-wetting child or older person with both innominates and coccyx in proper position." [**engineer**]

"The circuit of **electricity** is complete as proven by the complete arterial and venous circuit for the reduction of motor irritation."

"Some people say; 'It is such a nice place to talk, **eat** and visit'. Does an owl hoot and eat at the same time?"

"As life finds its general nutrient law in the fascia and its nerves, we must connect them to the great source of supply by a cord running the length of the spine, by which all nerves are connected with the brain.'" (**engineer**)

# F

"As a horse needs strength of the spur to enable him to carry a heavy load, so a man needs the **freedom** of all parts of the machinery power that comes from perfection of the body in order to accomplish the highest work of which it is capable."

"All long lived birds and animals, that live on but few kinds of **food**, should be a lesson for man not to eat and drink till the body is so **full** that no blood vessel can pass any part of the chest and the abdomen."

"I am simply trying to teach you what you are; to get you to realize your right to health and when you see the cures wrought here after all other means have failed, you can but know that the **foundation** of my work is laid on Nature's rock."

"A **fact** may and often does stay before our eyes for all time powerful in truth, but we heed not its lessons."

"As heat and motion have much to do as remedies, we may expect **fever** and pain until Nature's **furnace** produces heat, forms and converts its **fluids** into gas and other deposits, and passes them through the excretories to space, and allows the body to work normally again."

"**Fever** is a natural and powerful remedy."

"The Osteopath's **foundation** is that all the blood must move all the time in all parts to and from all organs."

"Why do you want to **fight** in time of peace? I told the multitude that in days of peace was the time to prepare for war."

"With us the **foundation** of life must be solidly constructed of stones of the highest grades of purity, or your house will lean toward the imperfect stones in the foundation; your building will bulge, crack, decay and fall down, and become simply a heap of ruins that will write the history of ignorance on the part of the architect and builder."

"When we have an infectious **fever,** that fever has possession of the whole body, and, by all rules of reason, will hold possession until it has completed its work."

"I know of no part of the body that equals the **fascia** as a hunting ground."

"The part the **fascia** takes in life and death gives us one of the greatest problems to solve."

"You see the **fascia**, and in your wonder and surprise you exclaim, 'Omnipresent in man and all other living beings of land and sea.'"

"If a thousand kinds of **fluid** exist in our bodies, a thousand uses require them, or they would not appear."

"What is the matter with your battery when you have **fever**?"

"If God made a man and made him liable to catch **afire** and made no provisions for putting out that fire He did not make a perfect man."

"In proportion to the velocity with which the heart brings the electricity that is generated in the brain, the temperature is high or low." (**fever**)

"I had great **faith** in my preacher and in my doctor. And I have not lost that faith. God knows that they did what they thought best."

"**Food** only provides **fuel** to keep the **furnace** warm."

"God is the **father** of Osteopathy, and I am not ashamed of the child of His mind."

"I want to drag both of your **feet** out of the ruts of allopathy, and place your hands upon the handle of the pump and get some water from the lymphatics, the cellular system of the lungs, or any other place in the human body, get the excretories all to work and put the **fire** out, like any sensible **fireman** would do if a city block were on fire."

"Be sure the **foundation** is level and all will be well."

"Let's be **finders** and **fixers** and not Pill-Peddlers."

"This heat (**fever**) never appears until the water supplying the lymphatics is very much exhausted."

"Lungs have **five** lobes, three on the right lung; and two on the left. Liver has five lobes, three on the right lobe and two on the left lobe. Nerves have five qualities; nutrition, sensation, motion, voluntary and involuntary. Nerves have five senses; seeing, hearing, feeling, smelling, and tasting. Since all principles differ in qualities or kinds of service, would it be amiss for us to inquire a little farther why the lungs and the liver are provided with five divisions each, if not to do five kinds of work, and different from all other kinds in many ways?"[17]

"Eat three conservative meals a day. Do not be a glutton! You can poison your system with too much **food** too often and of the wrong kind. Food is for energy only. As the body uses same, it should be replaced. When more food is added, you have cinders in your stomach and bowels."

"You will learn that the body is self-creative, self-developing, self-sustaining, self-repairing, self-recup-erating, self-propelling, self-adjusting, and in doing all these things on its own power, it will use only those things which belong to the realm of **foods**."

"When man is said to have **fever**, he is only on '**fire**', to burn out the deadly gases which a perverted, abnormal laboratory has allowed to accumulate by **friction** of the journals of his body or in the supply of vital **fluids**."

"An Osteopath who knows his business has no use for a speculum, no use for a steel spindle or sound in the treatment of **female** diseases."

"**Fevers** are effects only."

"**Fever** is electric heat only."

"**Fevers** of the fall and summer season are neither hotter nor colder than the fevers of the winter or spring."

"A study of the nature of **fevers** leads us to the spine."

"If God's judgment is to be respected, a **fit** [seizure] is the life-saving step or move, perfectly natural, perfectly reasonable, and it should be respected and received as divinely wise, because on that natural action which is produced on the constrictor nerves first, then the muscles, veins, nerves, and the arteries with all their centers."

"The oftener **fits** [seizures] come the oftener the nutrient part of the sensory system cries aloud in its own unmistakable language that it must have nourishment, that it may run the machinery of life, or it must give up the ghost and die. In this dire extremity and struggle for life, it has asked the motor system to suspend its action, use its power, and squeeze out any part of the whole body, though it be the brain itself, a few drops of cerebro-spinal fluid, or anything higher or lower, so it may live."

"The afflicted one is intoxicated. Here is where she gets a poisonous alcohol, and will never be relieved permanently until the 'wet towel' of reason has been slapped on both sides of the attending physician's head, so he can hear the squeezing and rattling of regurgitation, and the straining and creaking of the **fluids** in their effort to pass thru the diaphragm."

"When we eat and drink we do so because we are hungry. We do that many years before we try to reason why we grow from small to large-sized bodies, of bone and muscle." [**food**]

"We must have **facts** to build upon or our **foundation** will fall away."

"The **field** is already overcrowded with Doctors who for these hundreds of years have treated their patients by rule instead of reason."[18]

"It's the fellow who can **find and fix** the things that are wrong while the patient is still living, not after they are dead whose services will be in demand."

"It is important that you **find it** and it is just as important to know when you have **fixed it** and to leave it alone, nature will do the rest."

"The most any Physician can do for a patient is to render operative the **forces** within the body itself."

"Not until I have been tried by **fire** did I cut loose from that stupidity, drugs. Not until my heart had been torn and lacerated with grief and affliction could I fully realize the inefficiency of drugs. Some may say that it was necessary that I should suffer in order that good might come, but I feel my grief came through gross ignorance on the part of the medical profession."

"**Fever** is nature's method to burn up the refuse that the organs of elimination have failed to remove from the body."

"Every blood vessel is accompanied and controlled by **forces** suited to the system of blood supply."

"Allow me to say that I love the old Doctors for their **faithfulness**; I pity them for their universal **failure**. I know their intentions were good."

"Brute **force** is dangerous. Hands off unless you know your business."

"The Osteopath well knows that he must have two normally pure **fluids**, blood and nerve fluid."

"Electricity is called in as the motor **force** to be used in expelling all unkindly substances."

"The **fascia** is the place to look for the cause of disease and the place to consult and begin the action of remedies in all diseases, even tho it be the birth of a child."

"Nutrition must be in action all the time and keep all the parts well supplied or a **failure** is sure to appear."

"Remember the **fascia** is what suffers and dies in all cases of death by bowels and lungs."

"The **fascia** is universal in man and equal in self to all other parts, and stands before the world today the greatest problem, the most pleasing thought."

"**Fascia** is the house of God, the dwelling place of the Infinite, so far as man is concerned."

"The **fascia** gives one of, if not the greatest problem to solve as to the part it takes in life and death."

"This life is surely too short to solve the uses of the **fascia** in animal life."

"We have no need for tongs to let the monthly **fluids** flow easily from the womb. You must drop the tool idea." [**female**]

"You must know what a healthy woman is before you can think and act wisely with the woman who has lost her health." [**female**]

"I believe that more golden thought will appear to the mind's eye as the study of **fascia** is pursued than any other division of the body."

"The soul of man, with all the streams of pure living water, seems to dwell in the **fascia** of his body."

"We see in the **fascia** the **framework** of life, the dwelling place in which life sojourns."

"When you deal with **fascia** you are doing business with the branch offices of the brain, under a general corporation law, treat these branch offices with the same degree of respect."

"All nerves go to and terminate in that great system the **fascia**."

"It matters little with an Osteopath how hot or how cold a patient gets, his object of observation being in another direction that leads him to seek the cause of this **fundamental fermenation** [*sic*] and boiling of the **fluids** in the body."

# G

"What is the difference in cutting the Pterygium off your eye or cutting off a pig's tail? To cut off a Pterygium it will grow again as it is an abnormal **growth**, but to cut off a pig's tail it will not grow again as it is a normal growth."

"The better I am acquainted with the parts and principles of this machine-man, the louder it speaks that from the start to finish it is the work of some trustworthy architect; and all the mysteries concerning health disappear, just in proportion to man's acquaintance with this sacred product, its parts and principles, separate, united, or in action." [**God**]

"All abnormal **growths** and their effects follow obstruction to the normal flow of the fluids of the body. It matters not where the obstruction is, trouble follows. If we do not know this law, but use the knife, tongs, tweezers, and serums, we show that we do not know the producing cause."

"I would advise you to bathe your heads long and often in the rivers of divine confidence, and pray **God** to take care of you with other weak-minded people, who pretend to know that which they have not studied."

"Rely on your anatomy, physiology, and rub your heads, or deny the perfection of **God** and intelli-gence, and say, I am only Osteopathy in one pocket and pills in the other and none in my head."

"In sickness has not **God** left man in a world of **guessing**? Guess what it is that's the matter? What to give, and guess the results? And when dead, guess where he goes. I decided then that God was not a guessing God, but a God of truth."

"The laws governing the **growth** of vegetation **govern** animal bodies in a similar way."

"There is a natural demand for **gas** in all healthy joints of the body."

"Before pain begins at the joints, you are sure to find that all **gas** or wind has left the joints. Thus electricity burns because of bone friction."

"I did not believe **God** was a whiskey and opium doctor."

"The great Wisdom knows no failures and asks no instructions from inferior man.'

"Follow your **guide** and fear no danger."

"The people expect more than **guessing** of an Osteopath."

"Every **ganglion** on the great chain of the sympathetic nerve has a special and important function, but upon the superior cervical falls the greatest burden of responsibility."

"I want to emphasize **God**, and give to Him the intelligence of a God, a God to be respected and followed to the letter by the doctors of my school."

"The **gas** that forms in the stomach and bowels is formed from raw or crude materials that are taken into the stomach as nourishment."

"**Gas** seems to be native to space and how it is condensed is the question for astronomers to solve."

"We as chemists of good health, to succeed in curing our patients, must keep the **gas-making** machine in good mechanical condition to do laboratory work, or we will surely fail to cure or even relieve our patients."

"Digestion is food reduced to atoms of **gas**, both by chemical union and animal heat."

"The stomach is a finely constructed retort."

"The task for the wise man is to find and locate the machinery that does the work of converting the food into **gas**."

"Why does one's stomach blow off **gas** continually, while the other does not? This is a very deep, serious and interesting question."

"The greatest **gas** works of all, are the lungs which receive the lymph almost in the pure state with the venous blood for its highest refining process before it can go to the heart as living blood."

"We enter and close the whole process of forming blood thru the **gas** process of digestion, the only reasonable method of getting bread into the condition of living blood."

"Have we not great reason to believe that digestion is Nature's process of reaching matter that is to be converted to the finest **gaseous** atoms before it can be formed into blood."

"Since **God** is supreme intelligence, He did not leave out of the body anything necessary for the continuance of life."

"The **God** I worship didn't make such mistakes."

"Life is the **God,** the wisdom, the power and the motion of all."

"The possession of the human body by an infectious **germ** can only be immune by germicidal possession."

"Give freedom to the solar plexus and it will soon furnish a **germicide** that will drive the burglars from the system by the way of the lungs, the kidneys, the skin and the bowels."

"I quote no authors but **God** and experience."[19]

"I often think that death comes from poisons absorbed from diseased **gases** generated in the system. When the fluids of the body are formed, they are chemically pure, full of life, and should pass out and on for uses for which they are designed."

"I was a disciple of the 'old school' for many years and among its most faithful practitioners, until a better intelligence and a better understanding of **God's** provision itself led me to sever the ties that once held me blindly to drug medication."

"Farms are the tables of **God**."

# H

"Don't worry about massive **hemorrhage**—your index finger can stop any hemorrhage in the body."

"**Health** permits of no stoppage of blood in either the veins or artery."

"**Harmony** only dwells where obstructions do not exist."

"To find **health** should be the object of the doctor. Anyone can find disease."

"The **heart** is undoubtedly the 'King of all, Lord of all', the first in command, the last to yield."

"**Homeopathy** has reduced the dose in drugs, and in the same ratio has allopathy found it possible to get along with less of those deadly articles. Every step that drops even one grain of drugs develops mind that can see more Deity and less drugs."

"**His** works prove His perfection."

"We must avoid the dust of **habit**. We must so adjust our telescopes that we may set our compass to run to stars of greater magnitude, that shine from the breast of the exacting Infinite."

"Courage and good sense are the **horns** that scatter **hay** for the calves to eat."

"I love **Him** because **He** can put sight in your body, hearing, sense of touch, in fact all five senses and about five hundred other kinds of senses on top of them."

"I love **Him** because **He** is a photographer. Your mind is a sensitive plate, and every word that is said is photographed there, and when you want to look at them you raise up the glass; you call that memory."

"I cannot be **happy** and be idle."

"Nerves are the children and associates of one mother—the **heart**. She, the heart, is the wise form-giving power of life. She is life centralized for the use of each and all animals."

"**Hemiplegia** means, when divided, 'half" and 'I strike', or paralysis of one half of the body."

"On every voyage of exploration, I have been able to bring a cargo of indisputable truths, that all remedies necessary to **health** exist in the human body."

"I seldom stand when I can sit; I seldom sit when I can lie down."

"Remember the **head** can and does turn in the pelvis to suit the easiest passage thru the bones, while in the fluids of the amniotic sac."

"Learn to give treatments without distressing the patients more than necessary but if the patient is cured he will soon forgive one for **hurting** them."

"When encountering a very severe post partum [*sic*] **hemorrhage** with no facilities available grab the hair over the symphysis and give it a yank and the shock will stop the hemorrhage."

"An intelligent **head** will soon learn that a soft **hand** and a gentle move is the **hand and the head** that get the desired results."

"I want to insist on bringing to your attention the importance in treating disease of the **head**, of keeping the road from the **heart** to the brain open and in first-class condition for the passage and delivery of pure arterial blood to the head."

"Each organ must help to keep up the universal **harmony** by furnishing its mite of its own kind!"

"All that gives you life and **health** comes straight from **heaven**."

"If your patient has a **headache** or pain don't use a pigtail (**hypodermic**) but find the cause and remove it."

**Health** holds dominion over the body by laws as immutable as the laws of gravitation and so long as we obey the laws that make for health, one need have no fear of disease."

"The **heart** is the most perfect of all engines known."

"There is only one kind of **heat** (fever) in all nature."

"Man's **heart** is his engine, and from this Fulton borrowed his idea of the steamboat and Morse his thought of telegraphy."

"The **heart** is but a part of the general circulatory tree. It does not pull or push. It only gives the circulation its initial impulse. Therefore it is good or bad according to the disturbance throughout the entire circulatory tree, and the fellow that only learns enough about it to just listen to the patient's heart and tell them how badly it is crippled, isn't going to do very much for a patient with any kind of heart trouble. But the fellow who learns how to keep the limbs off the lines and assist Nature in keeping the fluids and forces moving to and from the heart on time will rescue many a poor devil that has been cast upon the scrap pile."[20]

"If you have any generalship you will evade anything like reporting that there is no **hope** for your patient."

"The **heart** the fountain of life is the organ in the human body which imparts the attributes of life and knowledge to the blood so that it can proceed correctly with all its work."[21]

"I do not need to learn the form nor physical actions of the **heart** but I want to know what attributes of life are located in the heart between conception and manhood."

"**Hypermobility**, or the condition in which the joints of the spine and lower limbs become loose, is an effect following the stoppage of nutrition to the nerves of motion."

"It matters little to me what is thought or said; give me a patient with a good **heart**, a good brain, with an open road between and I will give you a healthy person in a few days instead of the sick one who is laboring under some of these so-called mysterious diseases, in which the anatomical engineer fails to find any mystery but does find the results of stagnation of the fluids of the body, the effect of inhaling poisonous gases."

"I think much of the diseases of the **heart** are not of the organ but from a feeble supply of electricity that is cut off in the medulla or heart nerves between the heart and the brain. Why singing and roaring of the ears in heart diseases, if there is no waste of pectoral electricity?"

"With the best eye of reason we see but dimly into the breast of man which contains the **heart**, the wonder of man and the secret of life."

"Some evidence crops out now and then that ancient methods of **healing** were natural and wisely applied and crowned with success."

"As we dip our cups deeper and deeper into the ocean of thought we begin to feel that the solution of life and **health** is close to the field of the telescope of our mental searchlights and soon we will find the road to health so plainly written that the wayfaring man cannot err tho he be a fool."

"Any variation from perfect **health** marks a degree of functional derangement in the physiological department of man."

# I

"A man dreads to give up his old boots for fear the new ones will pinch his feet." [**irritate**]

"All patterns for all things are **imitations** of what is found in the constructed being, man."

Upon spanking a little boy and realizing it was unjust, Dr. Still said, "Don't cry sonny; go buy yourself some candy." [**ignorance**]

"I pray the Lord to keep my head combed with a fine comb, and get all the **ignorance** out of it, for then thou knowest the dandruff of laziness is rank poison to knowledge, success, and progress. It is the dust of hoggish meanness. Keep it off, O Lord.

Amen."

"The river of **intelligence** is just as close to you and yours as it is to me and mine."

"Rely on your anatomy, physiology, and rest your heads, or deny the perfection of God and **intelligence**, and say, I am only Osteopathy in one pocket and pills in the other, and none in my head."

"I have proven that the laws of the **Infinite** are all-sufficient when properly administered."

"To make the sick well is no duty of the operator, but to adjust a part or whole of the system that the rivers of life may flow in and **irrigate** the famishing fields. To irrigate too much is as detrimental as too little or not at all."

"Make yourself a child of **inquiry** and a student of Nature."

"By extensive study, I have formed in my head a perpetual **image** of every articulation in the framework of the human body."

"I believe all **immunities** are based on the philosophy or law of possession. Possession is nine points of the law and is just as good in contagious infections as in governments or any forceful possession of property or power."[22]

"Some say that it was necessary that I should suffer in order that good might come, but I feel my grief came thru gross **ignorance** on the part of the medical profession."

"The next step is to advance that belief to an **intelligent** understanding."

"If you want to be an **imitator**, study in a bath house."

"Both mules did not go up the hill, because one was pulling downward." [**ignorance**]

"Man's **ignorance** has made a condition for the knife."

"A big however can cover a vast amount of **ignorance**."

# K

"The Osteopath uses the **knife** of blood to keep out the knife of steel."

Dr. Still told of attending the daughter of an Indian chief in **Kansas**, and when the chief sat on the ground questioning him at length about her sickness when he finally had the Old Doctor cornered and forced to reply, "I don't know". The chief took his finger and made a circle on the ground and commented, "Indian know so much", then with a larger radius circumscribed a larger circle and said, "Medicine man know so much, outside this Indian knows as much as Medicine man."

"We want **knowledge**, we are willing to pay for it, we want all we pay for, and we want our heads kept out of the sausage-mill of time wasting."

"Do you know that each nerve fiber for its place is **king** and lord of All?"

"Osteopathy has but little use for the **knife**, but when no human skill can avail to save life or limb without the knife or saw then we are willing to use anything or any method to save that life."

"The **knife** should never be used until all nerves, veins and arteries have failed to restore a healthy condition of the body in all its parts and functions."

"Osteopathy is **knowledge**, or it is nothing."

"There are two very large and powerful rivers passing fluids in opposite directions over a territory that I will call the **Klondike** of life. This territory is bounded on the east by a great wall which according to the old books is called the diaphragm. I would advise the practising Osteopath to do some very careful panning up and down the rivers of the Klondike, for if you fail to find gold and much of it, you would better spend the rest of your life where reason dwelleth not. Ever remember that ignorance of the geography and customs of this country is the wet powder of success?"[23]

"I have no wish to rob surgery of its useful claims, and its scientific merits to suffering man and beast. My object is to place the Osteopath's eye of reason on the hunt of the great 'whys' that the **knife** is useful at all."

"I would advise all men and women to travel to the tree of **knowledge**, stop and take a sleep, and leave your burdens of life, for I am sure you will find a label that will tell you what limb has the fruit of success."

"I do not want to go back to God with less **Knowledge** than when I was born."

"We want to **know** to a certainty that the only hope to save life is in the use of the **knife** before we use it."

"The use of the **knife** in everything and for everything must be stopped; not by statute law, but thru higher education of the masses, which will give them more confidence in Nature's ability to heal."

"For many years I have made it my business to exhaust every other means of relief before I used the **knife**."

"The knowing how or the lack of **knowing** how to re-establish this natural law will make of you either a success or a failure."

"In all **kidney** diseases honey is very palatable as a diet. The more honey the patient would eat the sooner the spine and kidneys would get better."

"At what time was the man or woman born that knew and left on record a true and reliable **knowledge** of the renal capsule? We do not know whether that is the organ that makes our teeth, our hair, or generates a powerful acid by which lime is kept in solution, so as not to form stones and such deposits." [**kidney**]

"No record shows the exact time when man's first foot appeared on the earth. A **knowledge** of his advent might be profitable."

"This is the tree of **knowledge** in whose shade all persons have received that instruction that was necessary to each individual's success in life, without which no man ever succeeded."

# L

"Nothing looks **large** to us now. In the past a spoonful of castor oil assumed enormous proportions; to-day it does not; for it is seldom seen, and is in use only among the stupid."

"The life of the **living tree** is with the bark and superficial fascia which lies between the bark of the body of the tree; its periosteum."

"Let us assume that the **liver** is the abiding placenta of all animated beings."

"With a diseased **liver** we have perverted action which possibly accounts for impure and unhealthy deposits in the nasal passage and other parts of the body in their own peculiar form."

"Thus we can do no more than feed and trust the **Laws of life** as nature gives them to man."

"Diet, fresh air and exercise have largely aided me in the work of my **life**."

"Before you can go out into the world and fight the fight you must master human anatomy and physical **laws**."

"Turn the waters of **life** loose at the brain, remove all hindrances and the work will be done, and give us the eternal **legacy**."

"A fixed point, a **lever**, a twist, or a screw power, can be used and are used by all operators."

"To remove a bone or any substance from its position the mechanic seeks to find and make a fixed point, then he makes use of the principles of the **lever**, the screw or the wedge, and with his hands gets the movement desired."

"The most sublime thought I ever had in my life is concerning the machinery and the works as I found them in the human construction, faithfully executing all of the known duties and the beauties of **life**."

"The Osteopaths are the champions of natural **law**."

"As one delves deeper and deeper into the machinery and exacting **laws of life**, he beholds works and workings of contented **laborers** of all parts of the common whole—the great shafts and pillars of an engine working to the fullness of the meaning of perfection."

"We strike at the source of **life** and death when we go into the **lymphatics**."

"What we meet with in all diseases is dead blood, stagnant **lymph,** and albumin in a semi-vital or dead and decomposing condition all through the lymphatics and other parts of the body, brain, lungs, kidneys, liver and fascia."

"The human body is a machine run by the unseen force called **life,** and that it may run harmoniously it is necessary that there be **liberty** of blood, nerves and arteries from the generating point to destination."

"Our **lungs** are surely the half-way place between **life** and death."

"The brain flushes the nerves of the **lymphatics** first, and more than any other system of the body."

"Thus the system of **lymphatics** is complete and universal in the whole body."

"I believe the **law of life** is simple and natural in both respects if wisely understood."

"We strike at the source of life and death when we go to the **lymphatics.**" [*sic* repeated]

"Our science is young, but the **laws that govern life** are as old as the hours of all ages."

"The eye is an organized effect, the **lymphatics** the cause, and in them the principle of **life** more abundantly dwells."

"No atom can leave the **lymphatics** in an imperfect state and get a union with any part of the body."

"Do not wound the **lymphatics**, as they are undoubtedly the life-giving centers and organs, it behooves us to handle them with wisdom and tenderness."

"In death the **lymphatics** are dark, in **life** they are healthy and red."[24]

"A knowledge of Osteopathy will prepare you to bring the system under the rulings of the physical **laws of life**."

"The doctor who uses **liquor** should have his head cut off, as the brain cells no longer can function normally."

"Scientific osteopathic care from infancy to the grave will **lengthen** a man's **life**, while medical care will shorten same to a marked degree."

"We speak of **life**, but know of it only as we see bodies move by life back of the visible matter."

"Does Nature have a finer matter that is invisible and that moves all that is visible to us?" (**life**)

"**Life** is surely a very finely prepared substance, which is the all-moving force of Nature, or that force that moves all nature from worlds to atoms."

"Human **life** is eternal. We have no proof otherwise. Life enters the forest of flesh as man. It carries constructing wisdom and ability."

"The **Lord** never runs out of material."

"Each strand in the cord of **love** is so pure that the acids of time never corrode it."

"We get our knowledge by '**littles**', we should be willing to impart by the same measure."

"God's pellets of **life** are always full and never fail."

"If the **laws of the universe** are systematic according to kind, then we must observe and follow each system faithfully if we expect to change effects, because every change in cause gives a new effect. The universe is governed by that law. That law is **life**."

"The doctor has treated the effect and not the cause; therefore it has been necessary to make **laws** in their favor."

"I believe that at an early day we will be successful with **lung** diseases—in fact, with diseases of all organs of the body, in proportion to our acquaintance with the omentum and mesentery."

"When Harvey solved the circulation of the blood, he only reached the banks of the river of **life**."

"We get the **leavings** of the medical world, their incurable cases."

"Nature means wisdom, means mental ability; means business honesty, and we must not disobey its teachings." [**laws of life**]

"The **lymphatic** system is the universal system of irrigation."

"Let your **light** so shine before man that the world will know you are an Osteopath pure and simple, and that no prouder title can follow a human name."

"We must go to school about one-half our time, in order to cultivate and stimulate our mental energies sufficiently well to follow the ordinary business pursuits of **life**."

"You will find that the same natural **law** when obstructed that produces a condition or allows one to exist, reestablished, will take it away."

"It will be an essential part of your training. But keep in mind while it may tell you how much the house is on fire, it does not tell you what started the fire and what is keeping it burning." (**law**)

"Remember this, that while punching, wringing and twisting your patient who has **lung** trouble, unless you have a thorough knowledge of the location of the lung, its form, its nerve and blood supply, you are doing your patient no good, and yourself a great deal of harm by your failure to give relief."

"Keep the gates of **life** all open."

"According to every method of reasoning the **lung** comes in as the 'Great I Am' of **living blood**."[25]

"A word to the doctor, I want you to open both of your eyes and look me square in the face. Can you afford in treating disease of the **lungs**, to give your verdict and prescribe drugs or manipulations as a doctor of medicine, an osteopath, or masseur, without first carefully examining the pleurae in all divisions and knowing that their nerve and blood supply are perfectly normal?"

"When will a doctor advise that a child's **limbs** be let loose in order to be healthy?"

"The philosopher reasons that the universe is governed by the attributes of the substance known as **life**. We say, the **Living God**, and what are His attributes but the sum total of all knowledge to rule and govern all parts and principles that are governed by any **law** of intelligence."

"The **life** of one being is not sufficient to form another being."

"I can think of **life** in each person as the being who makes the body of man and places all organs under its system of perfect action, both mental and physical."

"**Life** in man itself is man and the body is the empire he controls. The region of the heart is his headquarters where orders affecting the whole living government, man's body, are given and received."[26]

"I think the **law** of the freedom of the nutrient nervous system is equal if not superior in importance to the law of the free circulation of the blood."

"The 'Pill Doctor' says, 'Dr. Osteopath you have not told us why the Negro is immune and the white man subject to **locomotor ataxia**."

"My opinion as a chemist, mechanic and philosopher is that all this bugaboo about syphilis being the cause of **locomotor ataxia** is without a shadow of reason that could be accepted by any man who reasons from effect to cause. To me, locomotor ataxia in most cases is the effect of mercury and should be treated accordingly."

"**Life** is a substance which fills all of the space of the whole universe."

"**Life** in danger, and can be saved by skill, not by force and ignorance."

"'Cleanliness is next to Godliness'. Turn the waters of **life loose** at the brain, remove all hindrances and the work will be done, and give us the eternal **legacy, Longevity**."

"One would say we **live** by wind and to cut it off we die."

"Finer nerves dwell with the **lymphatics** than even with the eye."

"The **lymphatics** consume more of the finer fluids of the brain than the whole viscera combined."

"The **lymphatics** form, finish, temper and send the bricks to the builder with intelligence, that he may construct by adjusting all according to nature's plans and specifications."

"In all our treatment do not wound the **lymphatics** as they are undoubtedly the life-giving centers and organs."

"A student of **life** must take in parts and study their uses and relations to other parts and systems."

"I believe that it is natural to build and destroy all material form from the **lowest** animated being to the greatest rolling world."

"I believe no world could be constructed without strict obedience to a governing **law**, which gives size by addition and reduces that size by subtraction."

"Each engine has a sacred duty to perform under the penal **law** of death to itself and all other divisions of the whole being, man."

"We can do no more than feed and trust the **laws of life** as nature gives them to man."

"A suitable place is necessary first to deposit the active principle of **life**, be that what it may. Then a responsive kind of nourishment must be obtained by the being to be developed."

"All the processes of **earth-life** must be kept in perpetual motion to cultivate and be kept in healthy condition or the world would wither and die, and go to the tombs of space, to join the funeral processions of other dead worlds. Thus you see all nature comes and goes by the feat of wisely adjusted **laws**."

"**Life** can only display its natural forces by the visible action of the forms it produces."

"By nature you can reason on the roads that the powers of **life** are arranged to suit its system of motion."

"Motion is the first and only evidence of **life**."[27]

"While the **laws of life** and their procedure to execute and accomplish the work designed by nature for them to do, is mysterious and to the finite mind incomprehensible, you can only see what they do or perform, after the work is done and ready for your inspection."

"I would advise the practicing Osteopath to do some very careful panning up and down the rivers of this Klondike, for if you fail to find gold, and much of it, you had better spend the remainder of your **life** where reason dwelleth not."

"Our first and wisest step to successfully combat all diseases would be to inhibit first the nerves of the **lymphatics**, then produce muscular contracture and cause them to unload their diseased contents, and keep them unloading until renovation is absolutely complete; leaving the lymphatics in a purely healthy state, and keep them in this condition at any period of the disease."

"I have thought for many years that the **lymphatics** and cellular system of the fascia, of the brain, the lungs, and the heart throughout the whole system of blood supply, do get filled up with impure and unhealthy fluids, long before any disease makes its appearance, and that the procedure of changes known as fermentation with its electro-magnetic disturbances, were the cause of at least ninety per cent of the diseases that we labor to relieve by some chemical preparation called drugs."

"Let the **lymphatics** always receive and discharge naturally, if so we have no substance detained long enough to produce fermentation, fever, sickness and death."

"In man's body have been prepared and united the two kinds of **life**, the celestial and the terrestrial, and the result is man and beast."

"All matter is **living** substance."

"No part is so small or remote that it is not in direct connection with some part or chain of **lymphatics**."

"**Life** is that force sent forth by the Mind of the Universe to move all nature, and apply our energies to keep that living force at peace by retaining the house of life in good form from foundation to dome."

# M

"When I look upon the work of Nature it doesn't work for a dollar and a half a day: it works for results only. God's pay for labor and time is truth only. If it takes Him a **million** years to make a stone as large as a bean, the time and labor are freely given and the work honestly done."

"A **mule** goes out in the woods, eats what is good for him and refuses what is not. A man should have as much sense as a mule."

"**Mind** is the supreme ruler of all beings, from the **mites of life to the monsters of the land** and sea. Thus we see a ruling principle without limit."

"Primitive man was a **mathematician**, not by collegiate process but by native ability. He did not have to take a course in a university to study chemistry, because of the fact that he was a chemist when he was born."

"Most of our so-called learned men of today stand upon heaps of **mental** rubbish."

"All the processes of earth life must be in perpetual **motion** to be kept in a healthy condition: otherwise the world would wither and die and go to the tombs of space to join the funeral procession of other dead worlds."[27]

"The Osteopath's **mind** is the knife to sever the cords of ignorance which bind the public to drugs."

"Learn that you are a **machine**, your heart an engine, your lungs a fanning machine and a sieve, your brain with its two lobes an electric battery."

"We must remember that the internal **mammary** is a very long artery beginning at the first rib and extending to the pelvis. Much good health depends upon its good work."[28]

"The explorer for truth must be a czar of his own **mental** empire, unencumbered with anything that will annoy him when he makes his observations."

"It is my intention, while I live, to prosecute with untiring energy the unfoldment of the best **methods** of giving relief in sickness, by bringing the afflicted from the abnormal to the normal as nature intended."

"If **mind** is a gift of God to man for his use, let him use it. A mind is not in use when doing no good."

"Biogen or dual life, means eternal reciprocity that permeates all nature. Thus we have a union of **mind, matter** and life or **man**."

"As a little leaven leavens the whole loaf, would not a little diseased blood disease the whole viscera?" [**matter**]

"An atom is the limit of inaction, to the point at which life rests in **matter**, because of its crudity."

"When **matter** passes beyond the degree of being atomized farther, then it is life and it acts and forms itself to suit the body of any being in the world."

"When **matter** ceases to be divisible, it then becomes a fluid of life and easily unites with other atoms, and is a mass or body of living matter and recrystallizes into the form given by the parent causes."

"In man's body have been prepared and united the two kinds of life, the celestial and the terrestrial, and the result is man and beast." [**matter**]

"We know life only by the **motion** of **material** bodies."

"That **self-moving principle** which we see in all animal bodies we call life, because we see them **move** independent of other bodies and forces."

"All visible **matter** is retired from labor to rest."

"All **motion is matter** in action."

"An explosive is **matter in rest,** and an explosion is **matter in motion**; so of motion is man."

"Life begins to unfold by explosions of lower orders of **material** life in **matter**. Thus all action marks the amount and quality of explosives used by the body that moves."

"What we call life is **matter** at labor, death is **matter** minus explosive ability and at rest."

"In man nothing is imperfect excepting his reason." [**mind**]

"There seems to be greater wisdom shown in his construction than in his reasoning powers." [**mind**]

"We find man a skilled workman, and not an atom of life, a living germ of protoplasm." [**mind**]

"Absolute evidence of purer and deeper reason than we have been able to present stands recorded on the faces of many valuable 'lost arts' which we have never been able to equal." [**mind**]

"We are living in a **mechanical age**. The body has been neglected by so-called scientists that have for past generations made it a sewage disposal plant for their ignorance of internal medicine."

"If the **mechanic's machine** is not running correctly he adjusts it. Why not apply it to the human body since it is likewise a machine?"

"The **membranes** which hold the organs of the body in place lengthen by heat and contract by cold."

"By nature you can reason that the powers of life are arranged to suit its system of **motion**."

"As **motion** is the first and only evidence of life, by this thought we are conducted to the machinery thru which life works to accomplish the results as witnessed in 'motion'."

"I have studied man as a **machine**. I am an engineer. Man the most complex, intricate, and delicate constructed machine of all creation is the one with which the osteopath must become familiar."

"As a skilled **mechanic**, (God), imperfection in forms of all parts was a word that He did not com-prehend, because His works never possessed a flaw nor fault in form."

"God **manifests** Himself in **matter, motion and mind**. Study well His manifestations."

"The human body is a **machine** run by the unseen force called life."

"I have no desire to be a cat, which walks so lightly that it never creates a disturbance. I want to be **myself**, not 'them' not 'You', not 'Washington', but just myself; well plowed and cultivated."

"Fill and keep the **magazine** of force and motion supplied with that which is chemically pure and needful to the building up of this wonderful structure, commonly called man."

"**Man** is the only animal that is helpless when he is born. A baby would starve within reach of its mother's breast. A newborn calf would find his dinner. A chicken knows a grain of wheat from a stone as soon as it hatches. Man is like a chicken in a shell, the shell breaks when he dies and he has the full attributes of his species."

"I began to look at **man**. What did I find? I found myself in the presence of an engine—the greatest engine that mind could conceive."

"To repair signifies to readjust from the abnormal condition in which the **machinist** finds it, to the condition of the normal engine which stands in the shop of repairs, first lining up the wheels with straight journals."

"If **mind** is a gift of God to man for his use, let him use it. A mind is not in use when doing no good."

"I looked around me and asked myself where were the patients we, the doctors, had been treating for disease? And I was compelled to answer, 'They are dead!' and it was then that I realized that something was wrong with **medicine**."

"The intelligence of Deity is unquestionable; His law unalterable. On this law is the science of Osteopathy founded, and after struggling for years under the most adverse circumstances it stands today triumphant." [**medicine**]

"Believing that a loving, intelligent **Maker of Man** had deposited in this body some place or through the whole system drugs in abundance to cure all infirmities, on every voyage of exploration I have been able to bring back a cargo of indisputable truths, that all the remedies necessary to health exist in the human body. They can be administered by adjusting the body in such condition that the remedies may naturally associate themselves together, hear the cries, and relieve the afflicted."

"Since the days of Aesculapius the delusion that has flourished is that **man** must swallow **medicine** to rid himself of disease."

"All **manipulators** are not Osteopaths any more than all butchers are surgeons."

"The **mind** has lost the quickening power of **mental** gratitude, and has grown so stupid by the purgative action of selfishness as to expel from his memory a desire to express to all persons, from the infant at the breast to the grave-dipping foot of the aged, by kindly words and deeds, to all persons who have ever thrown a rose, a crumb of bread, or a soft feather that would make his road easier, his heart happier, his mind more at rest, in my judgment is guilty of one of the most unpardonable offenses that the pen of man has ever recorded or the mind of justice could contemplate."

"The **mathematics** of heaven are perfectly trustworthy."

"This is my book with all directions, instructions, doses and sizes and quantities to be used in all cases of sickness, and with the beginning of **man**, in childhood, youth, and declining days."

"The **medical** doctors reason that the body has chemicals in it that have to be met with other chemicals or poisons."

"If you expect to be a successful **mechanic**, act like one who is governed by the square, plumb and level of reason, knowing just why such effects have been produced."

**Mind** by its unlimited skilled rules, governs and uses at will all forces and elements."

"The ability of the **mind** is shown by its power to rule and govern all forces wisely and to prepare, construct and **manage the motion** of this and all other worlds of the universe."

"Nature's object in fetal life is the production of a **machine** which when completed is sent forth for a purpose."

"The hour of birth is the beginning of intellectual conception when a new being, the intellectual **man**, begins to develop."

"To the **mechanic** all abnormalities are effects."

"All **mental** orders are based upon the favorable or unfavorable report of one or more of the five sensory sets of nerves."

"The five senses make their report to the superior ruler of the emotions which is **mentality**."

"Whenever **mentality** is not powerful enough to control the emotional we have the condition known as insanity."

"Your first position is that of a **master mechanic**, who is capable of drawing plans and writing minutely a specification whereby the engineer may know what a well constructed mechanic is in every particular."

"Our professional **men** are only imitators of one another."

"The length and width of the territory thru which the river of life (**mammary artery**) travels for the purpose of supplying organs, glands, membranes, and muscles is standing evidence to its importance to life."

"**Memory** calls up the past; reason sees tomorrow."

"**Man** represents the **mind** and wisdom of God to the degree of his endowments."

# N

"I have not only worked to relieve the sick, but I have had both eyes open all the time to find a defect in **nature's** work, its object, its plan, its specifications, its building and its engineering; so far I have failed to find a variation from perfection."

"**Nature** is a school of questions and answers, which seems to be the only school in which man learns anything."

"**Nature** never changes."

"When you have adjusted the physical to its normal demands, **Nature** universally supplies the remainder."

"No **nerve** can do its part unless it be well-**nourished**."

"The more we know of the architecture of the God of **Nature** and the closer we follow it, the better we will be pleased with the results of our work."

"When the **nerves** cannot take up **nutrition**, they will take up destruction and other elements which are detrimental to the process of nutrition and there is no other chance for relief except in unloading."

"I thought the swords and cannons of **nature** were pointed and trained upon our systems of drug doctoring."

"**Nature** applies to you the switch of pain, when her mandates are disregarded, and when you feel the smarting of the switch, do not pour drugs into your stomachs, but let a skillful engineer adjust your human machine, so that every part works in accordance with Nature's requirements."

"The most that any physician can do in treating disease is to render operative the **natural** forces within the patient's body."

"**Nature** has no apology to offer. It does the work if you know how to line up the parts; then food and rest are all that is required."

"Alcohol is rated in the pharmacopoeia as a stimulant but my observation is that it is a **narcotic** and the pharmacopoeia will be changed stating that alcohol is a narcotic." (It was changed in 1908).

"We must first acquaint ourselves with all its workings in the **normal** before we are prepared to comprehend or think intelligently of the meaning of the word 'abnormal'."

"Nothing is needed but plain, ordinary **nourishment**."

"The osteopathic mechanic must remember that **Nature** is a living critic and the answer must be yes or no."

"We must blend ourselves with, and travel in harmony with **Nature's** truths. When this great machine, man, ceases to move in all its parts, which we call death, the explorer's knife discovers no mind, no motion. He simply finds formulated matter with no motor to move it, with no mind to direct it."

"An osteopath is taught that **Nature** is to be trusted to the end."

"**Nature** would not be true to its own laws, if it would do good work with bad materials."

"Remove all obstructions, and when it is intelligently done **Nature** will kindly do the rest."

"**Nature** can and does successfully compound and combine elements for muscles, blood, teeth and bone."

"When we take up principles, we get down to **Nature**. It is ever willing and self-caring, self-feeding and self-protecting."

'Osteopathic machinists can go no farther than to adjust the abnormal condition, in which you find the afflicted. **Nature** will do the rest."

"The Osteopath must learn or know that no infringement can be tolerated in any part. **Nature's** demands are surely absolute, and require that the last farthing shall be paid in full."

"Beginning with lymph and finishing with fibrin and albumin, **Nature** prepares and bridges each step, and never fails to show success at the end of each effort."

"**Nature** and good sense are terms that mean much to persons who are used to set aside all else for facts."

"That **Nature** makes nothing in vain is an established fact in the minds of all persons whose observation has created in them a desire to reason. That having been my faith for many years, I tried to discover why Nature had made and placed in man's head so much fine machinery just to make a little ear wax."

"If **nothing** is made in vain, what is that bitter stuff made for? It is always there."

"**Nature** has never done any useless work or made anything in vain."

"It is my opinion that the ear wax should be kept in a fluid state. When in that state, the cells can more readily take it up and use it in the economy of life."

"We know that **Nature** would not be true to its

own laws if it would do good work with bad material."

"How can a carpenter build a good house out of rotten, twisted, or warped wood? If he can, then we can hope to be healthy with diseased blood."

"**Nature** has been thoughtful enough to place in man all that the word 'remedy' means."

"I have discovered that **Nature** is never without necessary remedies. I am better prepared today to say that God or Nature is the only doctor whom man should respect. Man should study and use the drugs of His drug-store."

"The Osteopath who succeeds best does so because he looks to **Nature** for knowledge and obeys her teachings: then he gets good results. He is often amazed to see how faithfully Nature sticks to system. A few years spent in the school of Nature teaches the Osteopath that principles govern the Universe, and he must obey all orders, or fail to cure his patients."

"We adjust the machinery and depend upon **Nature's** chemical laboratory for all elements necessary to repair, give ease and comfort while Nature's corpuscles do all the work **necessary**."

"Anxious **Nature** stands fully armed, and equipped and more than willing to execute all duties devolving upon her, knowing at the same time that obedience to these exacting laws is all that is known or accredited to them as success."

"Heat and cold receive their orders from the **neck**."

"We have two kinds of **nervous** systems, one that talks and the other that does not talk."

"The living person is the engine, **Nature** the engineer, and you the master mechanic."

"Man must be wise to know all about the neck, for by a twist of that **neck** we may become blind, deaf, spasmodic, lose speech and memory, and many other ills befall us."

"**Nature** has placed its manufactories above a given line in the breast, and develops the crude material below that line."

"Today is our day, **Nature** is our school and we must go by the pointings of the compass."

"**Nature** never made a philosopher. She made man to learn and act. Man can make of himself a philosopher or a fool."

"**Nature** splints a joint when there is pain in the articulation."

"**Nature** does not jump from the abnormal back to the normal. Step by step she retraces herself, that is why it takes time for the chronic cases to recover. See that your patients understand this."

"**Nature** is known only by the power of the fist or reason well applied."

"All **nerve** power issues from the heart and brain."

"Our work is done when we leave open the **nerve** channels to the perfect eye of **Nature's** inspection."

"0, Lord God Almighty! Thy wisdom is surely boundless, for I see that man must be wise to know all about the **neck**, for we find by a twist of the neck, we may become blind, deaf, spasmodic, lose speech and memory, and all that is known as the joys of man."

"If the **nerve** is not well **nourished** it will fail to execute its part for want of power—for by it all blood must move."

"**Nature's** demands are surely absolute, and require that the last farthing shall be paid in full"

"Which **nerve** slept while fat heaped up in useless piles in the body?"

"By the speed of man's ability we know and use

the comforts that **nature** holds in store for us until we call for and use them."

"When **nature** renovates it is never satisfied to leave any obstruction in any part of the body."

"**Nerve** force is not generated in the sympathetic system; the cerebro-spinal nerve force is conveyed to the ganglia by the rami communicates and in the ganglia is transformed into sympathetic nerve force. We might compare the ganglia to an electrical transformer."

"It is upon the smaller arteries that the sympathetic system has its greatest effect.'" [**nerves**]

"The schools of **Nature** are open and free to man. He can learn the lessons and become wise if he obeys the teachers; otherwise he leaves little and his knowledge is of little use all of his days."

"**Nutrition** must be in action on time, and keep all parts well supplied with power, or a failure is sure to appear."

"Every **nerve** must be free to act and do its part."

"Motor **nerves** must drive all substances to and sensation must judge the supply and demand."

"**Nature** moves by system in all her works. She succeeds in all because her plans are perfect. Her designs have an object as their day star, and with her eyes fixed on the plan the effect is seen to follow."

"A few years spent in the school of **Nature** teaches the Osteopath that principles govern the Universe, and he must obey all orders or fail to cure his patients."

# O

"The **Osteopath** has his own symptomatology. He seeks the cause, removes the obstruction and lets Nature's remedy—arterial blood—be the doctor; and when his patient is cured, he has in his system no blindly administered medicine with which he must contend."

"I think a writer on **Osteopathy** should speak from his own experience and keep his scissors out of the text books of the old schools which stand condemned as fallacious and untrustworthy in time of need."

"**Osteopaths** should never dread to meet the climatic or the diseases of the four seasons of the year."

"If he is an up-to-date **Osteopath** his hand is his thermometer; his hand his syringe. An Osteopath kills diphtheria worms with the club of reason dipped in pure arterial blood."

"An **Osteopath** should always remember that his highest attainment is that of the well-informed machinist and he should always feel that he is the judge who presides over the court of inquiry."

"If you can learn all of **Osteopathy** in four years I will buy you a farm, and a wife to run it and boss you."

"During the hottest period of the fight a musket ball passed through the lapels of my vest. Another minnie ball passed through my coat. Had the rebels known how near they were shooting at **Osteopathy**, perhaps they would not have been so careless."

"Pressure upon the symphysis will produce inhibition to the pudic nerve and relax the circular fibers of the **os**, thus hastening delivery."

"If **Osteopathy** is not complete in itself, it is nothing. Osteopathy walks hand in hand with nothing but nature's laws, and for this reason alone it marks the most significant progress in the history of scientific research, and is as plainly understood by the natural mind as the gold at eve-tide that decks the golden West."

"Stand by the old flag, **Osteopathy**, on whose fluttering folds are emblazoned in letters of glittering gold: 'One science, one Lord, one faith, and one baptism'."

"**Osteopathy** does not look on a man as a criminal before God to be puked, purged and make sick and crazy."

"**Osteopathy** is a science that analyzes man and finds that he partakes of Divine intelligence."

"We want no moderate **Osteopaths**."

"**Osteopathy** asks not the aid of anything else."

"**Osteopathy** stands pre-eminently above all things else."

"**Osteopathy** should be the lighthouse on which your eye must be continuously fixed."

"Let your light so shine before men that the world will know you are an **Osteopath** pure and simple, and that no prouder title can follow a human name."

"An **Osteopath** asks no favor of drugs."

"**Osteopathy** is God's law, and whoever can improve on God's law is superior to God himself."

"**Osteopathy** opens your eyes to see and to see clearly; it covers all phases of disease and is the law that keeps life in motion."

"The **Osteopath** reasons, if he reasons at all, that order and health are inseparable, and that when order in all parts is found, disease cannot prevail, and if order is complete and disease should be found, there is no use for order. And if order and health are universally one in union, then the doctor cannot usefully, physiologically, or philosophically be guided by any scale of reason otherwise."

"All **organs** belong to the brotherhood of labor, and they are commissioned to show perfect work and good health."

"An **Osteopath** should be clear-headed, conscientious, truth-loving man, and never speak until he knows he has found and can demonstrate the truth he claims to know."

"He must not be a blacksmith only, and only be able to hit large bones and muscles with a heavy hammer, but he must be able to use the most delicate instruments of the silversmith in adjusting the deranged, displaced bones, nerves, muscles, and remove all obstructions, and thereby set the machinery of life moving. To do this is to be an **Osteopath**."

"Our therapeutic house is just large enough for **Osteopathy** and when other methods are brought in, just that much osteopathy must move out."

"I do not claim to be the author of this science of **Osteopathy**. No human hand has framed its laws; I ask no greater honor than to have discovered it."

"**Osteopathy** cannot be imparted by books. Neither can it be taught to a person intelligently who does not fully understand anatomy from books and dissection."

"You wonder what **Osteopathy** is; you look in the medical dictionary and find as its definition, 'bone disease'. That is a grave mistake. It is compounded of two words, osteon, meaning bone, pathos, pathein, to suffer. Greek lexicographers say it is proper name for a science founded on a knowledge of bones. So instead of 'bone disease' it really means 'usage'."

"**Osteopathy** is a science."

"**Osteopathy** to me is a very sacred science. It is sacred because it is a healing power through all Nature."

"Vegetation builds forests, and cold builds mountains of ice to be dissolved and sent into the **ocean** to purify the water and to keep the brines from drying to powder, as salt."

"Let us not forget the assembling of **ourselves** together."

"No **osteopathic physician** has any business or any right to have an **Osteopathic** degree if he is incapable of correcting abnormal body structures."

"**Osteopathy** is as broad as the Universe."

"**Osteopathy** is an independent system and can be applied to all conditions of diseases, including purely surgical cases, and in these cases surgery is but a branch of Osteopathy."

"**Osteopathy** has no place for the masseur, but for the mechanics of first water, endowed by Nature and well qualified by practice."

"The **Osteopath** is the blacksmith at his anvil. The blacksmith proves his wit by his work. An osteopath shows his skill by the results of his work."

"No two **organs** are alike, therefore their responsibilities are different."

"**Osteopathy** is the practical knowledge of how man is made and how to right him when he gets wrong."

"**Osteopathy** walks hand in hand with nothing but nature's laws and for that reason alone it marks the most significant progress in the history of scientific research."

"The **osteopath** removes the obstruction, lets the life-giving current have full play, and the man is restored to health."

"Do **one thing** well and leave the rest alone."

"As an electrician controls electric currents, so an **Osteopath** controls the life currents and revives suspended forces."

"Not only must you be able to locate the **obstruction**, but you must have the skill to remove it."

"**Osteopathy** reflects Nature's cures."

"**Osteopathy** is a science; not what we know of it, the subject we are working with is deep as eternity. We know but little of it."

"**Osteopathic physicians** must be able to give a reason for the treatment they give, not so much to the patient, but to themselves."

"Unless you have something better to offer and can do the job better than it is being done, there is no excuse for your existence; and unless you teach it, preach it, and practice it, neither **Osteopathy** nor you will survive."

"Unless you keep in mind that neither **Osteopathy** nor its application to the patient can be passed around on a platter, you will not go very far in Osteopathy. You will be like the others that say Osteopathy needs a multitude of other things added to it."

"**Osteopathy** has come to stay without limit of time."

"**Osteopathy** is the greatest scientific gift of God to man."

"For every force in the body, there is an **opposing** force, the cause of the cause that is responsible for throwing the opposing force out of balance, must always be sought."

"The practical **Osteopath** must be very exacting in adjusting the system."

"**Osteopathy** is built upon the principal of debtor and creditor."

"The **Osteopath** must not fall back to the low plane of reason on which the masseur dwells."

"We are only tinkling symbols or sounding brass as **Osteopaths** until we can have reason at the beginning and the end of all our methods or efforts to cure the afflicted."

"An **Osteopath** must find the true corners as set by the Divine Surveyor."

"The first duty of the **obstetrician** is to carefully examine the bones of the pelvis and spine of the mother, to ascertain if they are normal in shape and position."

"I will give you a condensed rule of procedure in all normal cases of **Obstetrics**. With index finger examine **os uteri**; if closed and only backache, have Patient turn on right side and press hand on abdomen above pelvis, and gently press or lift belly up just enough to allow blood to pass down and up the pelvis and limbs. Relax all nerves of the pelvis at pubes."

"No breast should become caked in the hands of an **Osteopath**."[29]

"Tell the boys to keep it pure. Tell the boys to keep it pure." (Dr. Still made this statement at the last convention he attended. I think these words should be engraved on every diploma.) [**Osteopath**]

"This philosophy (**osteopathy**) knows no life nor death except thru the motion of blood and the inaction of that fluid, which contains life while in motion and death as to the effect of motion ceasing."

"I believe no world could be constructed without strict **obedience** to a governing law, which gives size by addition and reduces that size by subtraction."

"The **Osteopath** who succeeds best does so because he looks to Nature for knowledge and obeys her teachings then he gets good results. He is often amazed to see how faithfully Nature sticks to system."

"If you wound a tree in the forest it goes on thru all of the steps from the wound to gangrene and death. The **osteopath** must overcome similar wounds in the body by adjusting the parts in the locality of an organ injured. He is warned to keep the blood or sap in a condition to be delivered and appropriated."

"The science of **Osteopathy** is based on a system of reasoning that does not go beyond principles and truths that can be proven to exist in all of man's make-up, both physical and vital."

"All diseases of the organs of the abdomen should have the wisest methods of **osteopathy** exhausted before the knife is invited to take a part in this effort to rescue the life of the patient."

"There is an ever widening field for competent **Osteopaths**."

# P

"Carefully read up the nerve and blood supply of both lungs and the heart, because the lungs and the heart stand responsible for **perfect** health and every diseased organ depends on those two servants for recovery."

"I have found the ischia too close together in all cases of enlarged **prostate** glands that I have examined and treated in the past thirty years."

"If you have **polyps** or adenoid tumors of the nose would you take the tongs and pull out some nose this month and some more nose every other month or would you go to the nerve and blood supply and thru drainage regulate them?"

"We will have to reason that man is a machine of form and **power,** forming its own **parts** and generating its own powers as it has use for them. All powers are invisible and we see effect only. We know such forces to be abundant in Nature and life is sustained by them."

"I never go to sleep and forget to pray. I was taught my little **prayer** when I was young: 'I pray the Lord my soul to take'. Now I pray the Lord to keep my head combed with the fine comb and get all the ignorance out of it, for Thou knowest the dandruff of laziness is rank **poison** to knowledge, success and progress."

"Basic **principles** must at all times **precede** each **philosophical** conclusion. Principles to an Osteopath mean a **perfect plan** and specification to build in form a house, an engine, a man, a world, or anything for an object or purpose."

"Osteopathy walks hand in hand with nothing but Nature's laws, and for this reason alone it marks the most significant **progress** in the history of scientific research."

"We are to improve upon the failures of the **past** and give the **people** a science of healing with a **philosophy** that will feed the minds of the thinking."

"My object is to make the Osteopath a **philosopher**, and place him on the rock of reason. Then I will not have the worry of writing details, of how, to treat any organ of the human body, because he is qualified to the degree of knowing what has produced variations of all kinds in form and motion. I want to establish in his mind, the compass and searchlight by which to travel from the effect to the cause of all abnormality of the body. When you fully comprehend and travel by the laws of reason, confusion will be a stranger in all your combats with disease."³⁰

"A young **physician** should analyze and study his **patients** as they often are his best books."

"My **patient's** recovery was more to me than the dollars."

"Be careful and stop when your **patient** says, 'You hurt my neck'."

"I saw enough of Nature's **power** to adopt it as the best way to cure the sick and afflicted."

"If a man will die by means of **poisonous** medicine administered by way of his mouth, will he not also die from poisons generated in his own system by the law of fermentation and decomposition?"

"My father was a **progressive** farmer, and was always ready to lay aside an old **plow** if he could replace it with one better constructed for its work. All through life, I have ever been ready to buy a better plow."

"Two or more elements added together may cause **pain**."

"God has placed all the **principles** of motion, life and all has placed all he used in sickness, inside of the human body."

"Let us not be governed today by what we did yesterday, not tomorrow by what we do today, for day by day we must show **progress**."

"The Osteopath's duties as a **philosopher** admonish him that life and matter can be united, and that, that union cannot continue with any hindrance to free and absolute motion."

"We see the form of each world, and call the united action biogenic life. All material bodies have life terrestrial and all space has life, eternal or spiritual life." **[principles and philosphy]**

"Life terrestrial has motion and **power**; the celestial bodies have knowledge or wisdom."

"Biogen is the lives of the two in united action, that gives motion and growth to all things. Thus we have life terrestrial, or the **power** to move, and the wisdom from the celestial to govern all motions of worlds and beings, by union of the life of space and the life of matter."[31]

"If a seed is **planted** in the earth and it obeys both the terrestrial and celestial forces, then the results are a tree."

"A man's biogenic force, means both lives in united action to construct all bodies in form, with wisdom to govern their actions. Thus endowed, two beings or worlds." **[principles and philosophy]**

"When in contact, give wisdom and force to work out greater **problems** than either could accomplish alone."

"Biogen or material life of the two obeys the wisdom of the celestial mind or life." [**principles and philosophy**]

"Many of your **patients** are well six months before they are discharged. They continue treatment because they are weak, and they are weak because you keep them so by irritating the spinal cord."

"**Principles** to an Osteopath means a **perfect plan** and specification to build in form a house."

"The student of any **philosophy** succeeds best by the more simple methods of reasoning."

"I often think that death comes from the **poisonous** substances absorbed from diseased gases generated in the system. When the fluids of the body are formed, they are chemically **pure**, full of life, and should pass out and on for uses for which they were designed. No delays can be tolerated after they are prepared for use."

"Nature has furnished the flesh-eating animals, birds, and reptiles with **protective** musks of germifuge. Many can be smelled a mile or more. Any wild beast or bird can eat the most **putrefied** flesh of the mad-dog, small-pox or leper with perfect safety. They would be failures in Nature if they would take smallpox or hydrophobia and get wild and die. We would soon be without the buzzard of any other scavenger to clean the earth of **putrescence**."

"I want you to camp on the borders of the **pelvis** and stay there with your microscope, both in hand and head."

"**Piles** are caused by **pressure** on the bowels."

"**Perfection** is expected, must and shall be shown in every atom of arterial blood."

"I love God because His works are **perfect** and trustworthy, does not need any help and did not make man's stomach to be a slop-pail for any dopes or pills."

"The rattle-snake is an emblem of **poison**, and as all drugs are poisons, this conflict may be said to be the first conflict between Osteopathy and poison, in which Osteopathy came off victorious."

"Of the contents of the skull, one ounce is used for thought, the remainder generates **power** for the nerves."

"**Prophecy** is what can be seen by a cloudless mind, either of the past or future."[32]

"How many **persons**, observing ones, ever saw a sick goose on water tho the water be dirty?"

"Do you find any **principle** in heaven, on earth, in mind, in matter or motion, that is not represented by kind and quality in man's makeup?"

"When we take up **principles** we get down to Nature."

"When an Osteopath explores the human body for the cause of disease he knows he is dealing with complicated **perfection**."

"Still one part is just as great and useful as any other in its **place**. No part can be dispensed with."

"I want to emphasize to every Osteopath—never tell a patient he is in a bad fix, worse today than yesterday, or that he looks ill. I believe more **patients** suffer and die from such imprudence and fright than the world has ever dreamed of."

"I believe man made a mistake when he undertook to inject **poisonous** substances into the human system as a remedy for disease, instead of applying the laws of creation to that end."

"A horse may not have a beautiful body, but if he has 'get there' in his heels, he is the horse that wins the **prize**."

"Basic **principles** must at all times **precede** each **philosophical** conclusion."

"Our **professional** men are only imitators of one another."

"They spend many years in school because of a lack of native ability. This is our condition, and we must make the best of it."

"The great mass of **people** are like little robins; they open their mouths and gulp whatever the doctors advise. But they are vastly more ignorant, because the doctor is not giving food or anything that is constructive to body economy. Therefore, the doctors become enemies of their **patients**, as their **pills** are not food but too often—**poison**."

"When structural and **physiological** unbalance are not normalized, surgery is necessary to remove the **product** of abnormal structure and environment. When the diseased condition is removed; however, the field of destruction necessarily made by the surgeon's knife is dependent upon the normal **physiological** and structural environment to gain normal health."

"My object is to make the Osteopath a **philosopher**, and place him on the rock of reason. Then I will not have the worry of writing details of how to treat any organ of the human body, because he is qualified to the degree of knowing what has **produced** variations of all kinds in form and motion. I want to establish in his mind the compass and searchlight by which to travel from the effect to the cause of all abnormality of the body. When you fully comprehend and travel by the laws of reason, confusion will be a stranger in all your combats with disease."

"I am not conducting a school to teach a lot of **parrots**—not to turn out just another Doctor."

"**Purgative poisons** are taken up by the secretions conveyed to the lymphatics. To soften and wash out is the object of Nature. The lymphatics begin the work of washing out by starting action of the excretories and furnish the water to soften, which is injected into the bowels from the mouth to the extremities by a system of salivation."

"A **philosopher** knows he must submit to the conditions, and he is sorrowful in place of vengeful and vindictive, and all that is left for him to do is to trim his lamps and let the lights defend themselves."

"The Osteopath has great demands for his **powers** of reason when he considers the relation of diseases generally to the **pelvis** and this knowledge he must have before his work can be attended with success"

"Can a deep **philosopher** do otherwise than conclude that Nature has **planned** and placed in man all the qualities for his comfort and longevity? Or will he drink that which is deadly, and cast his vote for the crucifixion of knowledge?"

"If a man will die by means of **poisonous** medicines administered by way of his mouth, will he not also die from poisons generated in his own system by the law of fermentation and decomposition?"

"When all systems are cut off from a chance to **perform** and execute such duties as Nature has allotted to them, we have **prostration**."

"As a child I was taught that the difference between a doctor of law and a doctor of medicine existed in the fact that the doctor of law reasoned from cause to effect, which the doctor of medicine reasoned from effect to cause." [**philosopher**]

"Who has ever run up a white flag except the man who realized that he had no **power** to resist longer, no hope of victory."

"In all our labour to learn the hows and whys of **physiological** action, we only read the records of what man has seen after nature's machine has finished a tooth, an eye, ear, muscle or bone. He hears the music, but fails to imitate."

"I give you the **principle**, work it out for yourself."

"Where in all the vast array of literature—do we find a single sentence that would touch the facts that a depressed clavicle may cause a goiter, that a dorsal lesion is often responsible for stomach trouble — or that a slight dislocation of the hip may cause such intense pain in the foot, that **physicians** have often recommended amputation as the only cure?" [**principle**]

"The **public** does not think in terms of common sense. The Daddy and Mother Robin is [*sic*] trusted by their young because they look to them for food with the utmost confidence of their intelligence. Think!"

# Q

## Questions for Osteopaths[33]

"Are the human and animal forms complete as working machines?"

"Has nature furnished man with powers to make his bones; give them the needed shapes of durable material, strong in kind?"

"Does a section in Nature's laws provide fastenings to hold these to one another?"

"How will this body move, and how is the force applied and where?"

"Where and how is this force obtained?"

"How is it generated and supplied to these parts of motion?"

"What makes these muscles, ligaments, nerves, veins, arteries?"

"Are they self-forming, or has Nature prepared machinery to make them?"

"Does animal life contain knowledge and force to construct all of the parts of Man?"

"Can it run the machine after it has finished it?"

"By what power does it move?"

"Is there a blood vessel running to all parts of this body to supply all these demands?"

"If it has a battery of force, where is it?"

"What does it use for force?"

"Is it electricity? If so how does it collect and use this substance?"

"How does it convey its powers to any or all places?"

"How does the man keep warm without fire?"

How does he build and lose flesh all the time?"

Where and how is the supply made and delivered to proper places?"

"How is it applied and what holds it to its place when adjusted?"

"What makes it build the house of life?"

"Are the laws of animal life sufficient to do all this work of building and repairing wastes and keep it in running condition?"

"If it does, what can man do or suggest to help it?"

"Is this machine capable of being run fast or slow if need be?"

"Does man have in him some kind of chemical laboratory that can turn out such products as he needs to fill all his physical demands?"

"If by heat, exercise, or any other cause he gets warm, can that chemistry cool him to normal?"

"If too cold can it warm him? Can it adjust him to heat and cold?"

"If so, how is it done? Is the law of life and longevity fully vindicated in man's make up?"

# R

"My compass was **reason**; my test was that all truths do love and agree with all others."

"When you fully comprehend and travel by the laws of **reason**, confusion will be a stranger in all your combats with disease."

"When you are called to treat a case of **relapse**, I will say for the benefit of the operator that you have a case of fluid stagnation of the whole system."

"It is your eye of **reason** and your finger of touch that I exhort to be instant in season and out of season."

"Keep your mud valves open and your engine in such condition that you can move out of the hearing of theories and halt for all coming days by the side of the **river** of the pure waters of reason and be able to demonstrate that which you assert."

"I want to feel the branding-iron of **reason**, then I will know the truth by the depth of the burn."

"Now the doctor or bird-dog, can find quails of

**reason** in but one field that would lead him to the cause."

"**Remember** this, that a horse that is always hunting bogeys never finds a smooth road."

"In the highest lexicon of Osteopathy there is no word as '**rut**'."

"Don't accept anything as truth from anybody not even the old Doctor unless it filters through your God given **reason**."

"Now Lord we beseech Thee, once in a great while to pummel our heads with the hailstones of **reason**."

"If we wish to be governed by **reason**, we must take a position that is founded on truth and capable of presenting facts, to prove the validity of all truths we present."

"I did not navigate by the force of steam or wind, but by the great electro-magnetic battery of **reason**."

"The doctor of law **reasons** from cause to effect, the doctor of medicine reasons from effect to cause."

"When Nature **renovates** it is never satisfied to leave any obstructions in any part of the body."

"The doctor of Osteopathy has much to think about when he consults natural **remedies** and how they are supplied and administered."

"Our **road** is straight thru the woods. Old trees must fall, stumps must be taken out, trees of life and hope must be planted to declare the intelligence of the Architect of Life."

"It would be good advice never to enter a contest without your saber which is the purest steel of **reason**."

"By heat all metals melt. Acid must have oxygen to make them solvents of metals."

"I have never failed to find all **remedies** in plain view on the front shelves of the store of the Infinite."

"Nature is never without necessary **remedies**."

"God or Nature are the only doctor whom Man should **respect**."

"All **remedies** necessary to good health exist in the human body. They can be administered by adjusting the body in such condition that the remedies may naturally associate themselves together."

"A hen shows **results** by the worms she scratches out."

"It's never a question as to what the **remedy** or the treatment will do to the body, but what will the body do with the remedy or the treatment."

"**Reasoning** is the action of the mind while hunting for the truth."

"Absolute evidence of purer and deeper **reasoning** than we have been able to present stands recorded on the faces of many valuable 'lost arts' which we have never been able to equal."

"Is it not **reasonable** to suppose that the powers of the mind have also degenerated from some cause."

"In him nothing is imperfect excepting his **reason**."

"The statute is a money-making provision and when the people arise they are the law of the country."

"His patient is starving, correct the third rib."

# S

"The **stomach** itself is a **sac**. When filled to its greatest capacity, it irritates all the surroundings, and in return they irritate the stomach. Then it unloads naturally for relief."

"Disease of the nerves of the pelvis comes from pressure of the bowels and other organs of the abdomen and osseous disturbances. Thus we have a cause for '**morning sickness**'."

"We find by any method of reasoning that '**morning sickness**' is the result of poisonous fluids being taken up by the **solar system**, and that is the effort to get such poisons out of the system that makes vomiting necessary."

"Try your reason and see the **stomach** below sicken and unload its burden. Is this sickness natural and wisely caused? If this is not the philosophy of midwifery, what is?"

"Be careful not to let the engine deface or tear the door as it comes out."

"By getting **sick,** muscles become convulsed with force enough to easily push out the new engine of life out into the open space, by Nature's team, that never fails to deliver all goods entrusted to its care."

"**Structure** governs function."

"He should let his eye camp day and night on the **spinal** column."

"All God's works, **spiritual** and material, are harmonious. His laws of animal life was absolute. So wise a God had certainly placed the remedy within the material house in which the spirit of life dwells. With this thought I trimmed my sails and launched my craft as an explorer."

"You find all men are **successes** or failures. Success is the stamp of truth. I will say all men who fail to place their feet on the dome of facts do so by not sieving all truth and throwing the faulty to one side."

"**Surgery,** manipulative treatment with or without instruments, distinguished from the practice of medicine, the administration of drugs."

Throw of your goggles and receive the rays of **sunlight** which forever stand in the bosom of Reason."

"The **seeker** of Truth is a man of few words and they are used by him only to show truth and facts he has discovered."

"Our **school** was created to improve on the past. Let us keep step with the music of progress. Read the charter of your school every night before you go to bed. I say 'improve' on old theories."

"Do **substances**, beings, animals, trees, and **stones** throw off an incubating vitality of their own? Can this life substance be conveyed to another body over a conducting wire, or is conveyed by the atmosphere? Is there not a life-giving force common to all nature, and when that force passes from a diseased human to another, does it not show by its action that it is a living substance?"

"Go to the **spine** and ribs only. If you do not know the power of the spinal nerves on the liver to restore health, you must learn or quit because you are only an owl of hoots, more work than brain."

"The osteopath who keeps his eye on the **science** and not on the almighty dollar, will be able to control all forms of disease."

"He who talks much, does little, and hates his successful brother or sister, because they have succeeded by perseverance, which he has failed to reach thru laziness and **stupidity**, will never succeed in anything."

"From occiput to coccyx you must know right from wrong or the results will not give **satisfaction**."

"The **solvent** powers of life dissolve all fluids and solids from blood to bone."

"Osteopathy is a **science** that analyzes man and finds that he partakes of Divine intelligence. It acquaints itself with all His attributes."

"**Sickness** is caused by the stopping of some supply of fluid or quality of life."

"No other **schooled** physician is capable of maintaining normalization of structure excepting an osteopathic physician."

"Treat the **spine** first and name the disease second. You will have time to go home and study or get consultation."

"Most doctors have five **senses**. Too many lack the sixth sense or horse sense."

"The **scientist** is only an ignorant man well fed with experience."

"God did not make man's **stomach** to be a slop-pail for any dopes or pills, big or small."

"Osteopathy has the highest respect for the science of **surgery**, which has been recognized as a science in all ages."

"The osteopath should remember that sensible **surgery** is a part of Osteopathy and his opinion if correct is good and if not correct will condemn his knowledge of cause and effect."

"The man who **succeeds** does more than follow a theory."

"Does order and **success** demand thought and cool-headed reason?"

"Pull the hair over the **symphysis** which will cause the womb to contract by irritation."

"We are warranted to conclude that Nature at will can and does produce the **solvents** which may be necessary to melt down deposits of fiber, bone or any fluid or solid found in the human body. If we grant this law, we must acknowledge an Infinite and perfect power to plan and execute its designs, compounding and creating any and all kinds of chemical substances to dissolve to the lowest order of fluids, which approach very closely the gaseous conditions of solids, previous to applying the renovating forces which must come in due time and carry away all dead, useless, and obstructing deposits, previous to inviting the corpuscles of construction to take possession." [34]

"**Success** is the reward of personal effort and confidence in self to solve all problems of life."

"Our great dinners are only slaughter-pens of show and **stupidity**."

"Life in danger, can be **saved** by skill, not by force and ignorance.

"Never **surrender**, but die in the last ditch."

"You should let your eyes rest day and night upon the **spinal** column."

"The **schools** of Nature are open and free to man."

"A **student** of life must take in all parts and study their uses and relations to other parts and systems."

"He who treats symptoms is the man who fights disease with specific and if intelligent and honest he will say, 'No **specific** has ever been found for any disease'."

"Osteopathy to me is a very **sacred** science. It is sacred because it is a healing power through all Nature."

"Local **shocks** affect the whole system, the nerve and blood supply to every part of the body. They disable and confuse the secretory and excretory systems and the fluids retained become deadly poisons."

"Our **schools** are not intended to use the greatest number of drugs that are allotted to man."

"You have as little use for old **symptomatology** as an Irishman has for a cork when the bottle is empty!"

"**Success** in any work will show the foundation on which the successful man and woman stood and without which no one can hope to succeed."

"I have only gotten the squirrel's tail out of the hole in the tree, and that it was up to us, his graduates, to 'dig on' and pull the remainder of the **squirrel** out of the hole."

"**Success** is the stamp of truth."

"Osteopathy is **surgery** from a physiological standpoint."

"I want men and women to **study** Osteopathy who reason and think for themselves."

"Keeping in mind the Osteopathic concept, the human body does not function in **separate** units, but only as a harmonious whole, and the fellow who masters it as such, will find that he is the Specialist of all Specialists, and that is a life-time job for any man or woman."

"**Symptomatology** is very wide and wise in putting this and that together and giving it names, but fails to give the cause of all abnormal lesions."

"Our **science** is young but the laws that govern life are as old as the hours of all ages."

"**Structure** on tension moves at its weakest point."

"Mr. **Spinal** Column and Mrs. Spinal Chord [*sic*] and their children, the nerves. Mr. Spinal Column goes on a 'bender' on Saturday night and, as was always the case, the greatest sufferers were the wife and the children. And so Mr. Spinal Column is brought before the Judge Heart and the jury (lungs) on Monday morning for the reckoning."

# T

"We often speak of **truth**. We say great truths, and use many other qualifying expressions. But no one truth is greater than any other truth. Each has a sphere of usefulness peculiar to itself; thus we should treat with respect and reverence all truths, great and small."

"I propounded to myself the serious question: 'In sickness has not God left man in a world of guessing'? Guess what is the matter? What to give, and guess the results? And when dead, guess where he goes. I decided that God was not a guessing God, but a God of **truth**."

"The original **thinker** on any subject cares nothing for so-called authority either of the past or the present."

"I am a lone **thinker**. I seldom speak for the multitude."

"It is the little **things** that are the big things in the Science of Osteopathy."

"Life is **truth** to you in proportion to what you know about it."

"God's pay for labor and **time** is **truth** and truth only."

"We can do no more than to feed and **trust** the laws of life as Nature gives them to man."

"If a **tumefaction** appears in one side and not in the other, why is it in the one side and not the other?"

"The **time** has come for practical man to lay down all understandable theories and prove what he says."

"If you were consulted on a case of enlarged **tonsils**, would you take your knife out of your belt, whack them off and throw them away or would you go to the atlas and axis as a sensible engineer and give nature a chance to reduce the **tonsil** to its normal condition."

"The instruments that I use in my laboratory when seeking for the cause and relief of **typhus** fever are spades, pitchforks, water and fire to dispose of all filth."

"I first saw the **tracks** of God in the snow of time. I followed them."

"**Tradition** has been the everlasting parent of tyranny."

"As we dip our cups deeper and deeper into the ocean of **thought** we begin to feel that the solution of life and health is close to the fields of the **telescope** of our mental searchlights and soon we will find the road to health so plainly written that the wayfaring man cannot err tho he be a fool."

"**Truth** has no cause to fear opinions. It wants no flattery. It neither loves nor hates. It is food and comfort."

"A **truth** is like a machine made for a purpose. All parts must be in place, and power applied to suit, or that machine fails to perform the service for which it is designed, and the object is lost if this is not done."

"We often speak of **truth**. A truth is the complete work of Nature, which can only be demonstrated by the vital principle belonging to that class of truths. Each truth or division as we see it can only be made known to us by the self-evident fact, which this truth is able to demonstrate by its action."[35]

"We are dealing with the omnipresent nerve principle of animal life, I will tell you this one serious **truth**. To treat the spine more than once or twice a week and thereby irritate the spinal cord will cause the vital assimilation to be perverted and become the death producing execution by effecting an abortion of the living molecules of life before they are fully matured and while they are in the cellular system, lying immediately under the lymphatics."

"I hate a hen that sits on a nest that has no eggs in it just because her grandmother sat there. If she sits on nothing but rotten eggs, what will she get but rotten chickens like the rotten virus Jenner put under his hen of reason a hundred years ago.'

"I want the man who wishes the work that is done by the organs or contents of the abdomen known, also to know the danger of ignorance, and that wild force in treating the abdomen cannot be **tolerated** as any part of this sacred philosophy."

"**Tumefaction** is only the natural effect that follows or appears in the abdomen or pelvis when lymph is stopped in its natural channels in any organ or part of the viscera."

"**Timidity** takes possession of us only when we are at a loss to judge of the end from the beginning."

"Ages have passed yet the people sicken, suffer, recover or die, and by habit or tradition we still follow the unsuccessful practice and methods of the old **theories**."

"The man who is a competent engineer of the human body should not allow **tumors** to form and because of his lack of knowledge of cause and effect say that he does not know the cause of their production."

"Let your mind penetrate to the remotest period of **thought** by the **telescope** of reason."

"It doesn't matter so much the name of the disease, the principal thought of the Osteopathic physician is to **treat** the spine, know how to normalize structure; function will take care of itself."

"When your machine does not run you take it to a mechanic, not to a chemist. Why do we have so many fools in the world? Take the 'H' out of thinker and you have **tinker**. Who wants a tinker for a physician?"

"This is a war not for conquest, popularity or power. It is an aggressive campaign for love, **truth** and humanity."

"I felt I must anchor my boat to living **truths** and follow them, wheresoever they might drift."

"The **thoughts** of God himself are found in every drop of your blood."

"The earth goes round the sun on **time** to a minute. If she should stop to **talk** politics, it would jerk your head off."

"Diseases of the **tonsils** are an effect of pressure and constriction."

"Fundamentals of **truth** are only obtained by studious attention to business."

"A **truth** is only a hopeful supposition if it not supported by results."

"Attend to one **thing** at a time, and that one thing all the time."

"Don't fool away your **time** fumbling to 'stimulate' and 'inhibit'."

"The **thinker** reduces his thoughts to practice, and cuts the grain, leaving it in condition that a raker is needed to bunch it, previous to binding."

"We can never improve old **theories** to the degree of **truths**. They are not based on facts. When we turn our eyes and look back for truths, back from Nature, we only behold the dark clouds of dying theories, without a single friend to mourn their loss."

"In Osteopathy we have the **tree** of life, and the living man in it."

"Our science sees him, our science has proven him to be a living man proven him to be the work of a living God, a wise God, whose words are alive and show wisdom in form and purpose."

"All is guess-work, whose father and mother are '**tradition** and ignorance."

"Does it not throw hot shot and shells of **thought** into man's famishing chamber of reason."

"**Talk** is talk, but the biscuit speaks for the cook."

"Here I want to emphasize that the word **'treat'** has but one meaning, that is to know you are right, and do your work accordingly."

"The ancients did much **thinking**. Great minds existed then, as is evidenced by the architecture displayed in the buildings of the temples and pyramids."

"In philosophy, chemistry and mathematics we have living facts of their intelligence."

"**Temperature** regulates the motion of the universe and all bodies therein. Life in motion is an effect of temperature just above 90 degrees F. Death is inaction, a lack of heat or motion."

"We arrive at **truth** only by the powerful rules of reason, the philosopher has shouted from the house tops during all these ages. He adjusts his many supportable causes, and adds to and subtracts from until he arrives at a conclusion based upon the facts of his observations. We must know the principles that exist in substances and seeds by which, when associated with proper conditions, that powerful engine known as 'animal life' gives truth, with fact and motion as its vouchers."

# U

"Parts and **uses** of the human body today are to us as little understood as electricity was at any time."

"The **unity** and oneness of the body."

"In **urinalysis** you are told, 'here is fat', 'here is sugar', 'here is iron', 'here is pus', 'here is albumin', and 'this is diabetes', 'this is Bright's disease', but no suggestion is handed to the student's mind to make him know these numerous variations from the normal urine are simply effects, and the diaphragm has caused all the trouble."[36]

"I find in man a miniature **Universe**."

"As you advance in your **understanding**, you will find it is always the deeper structures that are responsible in keeping the parts in lesion when they have once formed, and no amount of massaging of the superficial tissues will adjust a bony lesion."

# V

"We see wisdom just as much in the **venous** system, as in the arterial."

"Ladies and gentlemen you are getting lectures on **venereal** diseases against my wishes. The lecturer calls this gonorrhea, that is a nicer name but it simply means a good old fashioned clap, and I don't want my graduates, men and women to go out to be clap doctors, do I make that clear? I don't like the good name of Osteopathy to be linked up with such a disease. Just tell such patients to keep their pants buttoned as they should and keep out of that mess for you don't want a reputation of being a doctor who builds up his reputation on that type of disease. Is that plain, do I make my position clear?"

"God provides water buckets and water for the **veins**."

"I would not antagonize the popular belief in the efficacy of **vaccination** but do most emphatically combat the insertion into the human body of putrid flesh of any animal."

"See the busy mind of God rejoice at the beautiful work of his machinery, cutting and designing forms for fowl of the air and fish of the sea."

"Animals, fish and fowl, angels and worlds, are atoms of which you are composed."

"Some of us do not have to go to sleep to see **visions**."

"To do justice to gynecological service you must be a work hand in the navy yard of life, and must examine the whole **vessel** when she comes to dock for repairs, it is not necessary to look at the bottom of this ship all the time. Look at all parts with equal energy. Go over the whole hull and see if holes or cracks let water come into the hull."

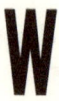

" '**Wind**' and **Wisdom** never blend."[37]

"The Great **Wisdom** knows no failures and asks no instructions from inferior man."

"When you get out in the field—if you are not going to be **willing** to take off your coat, roll up your sleeves and go to work, you had better pack up your books and go home now."

"To know the spinal column from beginning to end is **wisdom** that we must have or fail."

"A congestion following changes of weather from hot to cold, dry to wet or damp, is a **wound**."

"**Woman** is finer principled than man, she is sensory, man motor. He is motor, she is intellectual."

"Both the stomach and the **womb** receive and distribute nourishment to sustain animal life. Both get sick; both vomit when irritated and discharge their load by the natural law of 'throw up' and 'throw down'."

"The one is the upper stomach that takes coarser material and refines the unrefined substances, and keeps the outer man in form and being. The other contains the inner man or child, and by the law of ejection, when it becomes an irritant, it is thrown out by the nerves that govern the muscles of ejection."[38]

"I am at a loss to know why so much **wind** is taken into the body just to blow out. One would say we live by the wind, and to cut it off we die."

"I asked of my own reason if there was not a cloud of **water** in the human body that could be caused to drop its dews, put out the fires of fever, and save the forests of life that were being burned every fall season."

"I **want** to draw your attention to the fact that there is no method known by which electricity or magnetic forces can be weighed."

"Use no man's opinions; accept his **works** only."

"I love God because I cannot find any contradictions when I examine His **works**."

"**War** comes to settle a difficulty thru which the brain cannot see."

"The liver stands today one of the **wonders** to him that tries to understand."

"I **worship** a respectable, intelligent and mathematical God."

"The **wheels** of your back are cramped, just as your **wagon** cramps if you make a short turn."

"**What** has been the procedure in human life? Has it not been to select the strong and healthy male and drive them out to the field of battle to destroy a million or more of other strong men?"

"There seems to be a greater reason shown in Man's construction than in his reasoning powers." [**Wisdom**]

"We find man a skilled **workman**, and not an atom of life, a living germ of protoplasm."

"Thus to construct **wisely** is natural to all beings."

"Use your brain, your knowledge of anatomy and your powers of reason. Throw away your cough drops to the dogs." [**Wisdom**]

"I never advise him who knows enough." [**Wisdom**]

# Original Bibliography

*Philosophy of Osteopathy*, Andrew T. Still

*Academy of Applied Osteopathy*, Year Book, 1948

*Osteopathy Research and Practice*, Andrew T. Still

*Autobiography of Dr. Still*, Andrew T. Still

*Principles and Practice of Osteopathy*, Andrew T. Still

*Philosophy and Mechanical Principles of Osteopathy*, Andrew T. Still

# Revised Bibliography

Still AT. *Philosophy of Osteopathy*. Kirksville, MO: A.T. Still; 1899.

*Academy of Applied Osteopathy*, Year Book, 1948. (Note the Academy of Applied Osteopathy was renamed the American Academy of Osteopathy in 1970.)

Still AT. *Osteopathy Research and Practice*. Kirksville, MO: The Journal Printing Co; 1910.

Still AT. *Autobiography of Andrew T. Still with a History of the Discovery and Development of the Science of Osteopathy*. Kirksville, MO: published by the author; 1897.

Still AT. *The Philosophy and Mechanical Principles of Osteopathy*. Kansas City, MO: Hudson-Kimberly Pub Co; 1902. (Note: Although published in 1902, copyright year was 1892 by Andrew Taylor Still).

# Notes

## A

1. **Page 16, "My advice is to let your object be to keep out of papers…"**

   This excerpt is from *Osteopathy, Research and Practice*, Chapter "Osteopathy and the Solidity of Its Foundation," page 509, paragraph 903.

   To know your business (Osteopathy), you must know you are a part of nature. Follow your experience with nature's laws instead of keeping your head too much in books and paperwork. As you do good work (God's work, Nature's work, the work of the Stillness), the patients will follow.

2. **Page 17, "Arterial motion is normal during all ages…"**

   This excerpt is from *The Philosophy and Mechanical Principles of Osteopathy*, Chapter II "Some Substances of the Body," in the section "The Brain," page 41. The lines that follow add more depth and clarity to this statement:

"Arterial motion is normal during all ages, from the quick pulse of the babe's arm to the slow pulse of the aged. At advanced age the pulse is so slow that heat is not sufficiently generated by the nerves, whose force is not great enough to bring electricity to the stage of heat. All temperature, high and low, surely is the effect of active electricity—*plus* to fever, *minus* to coldness. When an irritant enters the body by the lungs, skin, or in any other way, a change appears in the heart's action from its effect on the brain to a high electric action. That burning heat is called fever. If *plus*, we may have a violent type, as in yellow fever; if *minus*, we may have low grades, as in typhus and typhoid fevers, and so on through the list."

# B

3. **Page 19, "The brain of man was God's drugstore…"**

   This line is from the *Autobiography of Andrew T. Still*, Chapter XIV, in the section "A Disturbed Artery and the Result," page 219.

4. **Page 21, "The first step in Osteopathy is belief in our own body."**

   This quote was recorded by Freshman HH Gavett, January 1896, and was included in the *AAO Yearbook*, 1948, pages 48-49, as referenced by John Lewis is his book *A.T. Still: From the Dry Bone to the Living Man*, 2012, page 156. Here is a continuation of that narrative:

   "The next step is to advance that belief to an intelligent understanding. You will learn that the body is self-creative, self-developing, self-sustaining, self-repairing, self-recuperating, self-propelling, self-adjusting and does all these things on its own power. It will use only those things which belong to the realm of foods.

I want to impress upon you in the beginning of your study of Osteopathy with the things that you must know to make a success of it:

First, Osteopathy is not a system of movements [techniques];

Second, neither Osteopathy nor its application to the patient is something that can be passed around on a platter. One must delve and dig for it themselves;

Third, its application to the patient must be given by reason and not by rule. Osteopathic physicians must be able to give a reason for the treatment they give, not so much to the patient, but to themselves.

Neither am I operating a school to teach a lot of parrots, or turn out just another doctor. The field is already overcrowded with those who for these hundreds of years have treated the patients by rule rather than reason."

5. **Page 21, Never mind what the book says..."**

The source for this line could not be found. There is a similar story from the Charles E. Still (CES) collection, in the Museum of Osteopathic Medicine, 1997.04.119, 34-, as researched by John Lewis in his book, A.T. Still: From the Dry Bone to the Living Man, 2012, pg 256. The account says that Dr. Still comes to the classroom and says, "Boys and Girls, I'm going to draw you a pig" and draws a turkey, instead. "You read in your textbooks that pneumonia is such and such and so and so. Maybe it is. But you look for yourselves, under osteopathic teachings, and see everything, not just what the book says. It is a turkey, not a pig. You never find it if you don't look for it, but if you look for it you will find it. If you treat the case according to what the book says [expecting to find a pig], you will get what the book promises you which is not much. If you treat what you find [a turkey], as osteopathic physicians you should be able to cure your case. That is the science of osteopathy. To take no man's word for it. You examine the body as an engineer, and the body shows you what to do, what needs to be done."

6. **Page 23, "Remember that during childbirth the bladder…"**

   This line is from *Osteopathy, Research and Practice*, Chapter "Menopause," page 295, paragraph 515.

   William Garner Sutherland, D.O., also said that "Sag rhymes with drag; and sags and fascial drags lead to chronic rags!" from the 1954 Osteopathic Cranial Academy News Letter, Vol. 8, No. 2, November, 1954, In Memoriam for Dr. William Garner Sutherland (1873-1954).

7. **Page 24, "The brain flushes the nerves of the lymphatics first…"**

   This line is from *Philosophy of Osteopathy*, Chapter VI "The Lymphatics," in the section "Nature's Solvents," page 66.

   Osteopaths have worked with the brain lymphatics for over a century. However, it was not until 2012 that researchers elucidated a lymphatic system of the brain which they called glymphatics (for glial-lymphatics). Scientists have also re-discovered the meningeal lymphatic system, which was described at the end of the 18th century by the anatomist Paolo Mascagni but was "forgotten". Both the glymphatics and meningeal lymphatics are functionally connected. These brain lymphatic systems help clear wastes and metabolites as well as distribute nutrients and neurotransmitters.

   Jessen NA, Munk AS, Lundgaard I, Nedergaard M. The Glymphatic System: A Beginner's Guide. *Neurochem Res.* 2015 Dec;40(12):2583-99.

Licastro, E., Pignataro, G., Iliff, J.J. et al. Glymphatic and lymphatic communication with systemic responses during physiological and pathological conditions in the central nervous system. *Commun Biol* 7, 229 (2024).

Da Mesquita S, Fu Z, Kipnis J. The Meningeal Lymphatic System: A New Player in Neurophysiology. *Neuron.* 2018 Oct 24;100(2):375-388.

8. **Page 25, "Slaves and savages…"**

    This excerpt is from *The Philosophy and Mechanical Principles of Osteopathy*, Chapter II "Some Substances of the Body, in the section "Thought Implies Action," pages 41-42. Here, he describes that chronic overthinking can lead to stroke and a stoppage of nutrition to the brain, hence causing hemiplegia. Dr. Still notes that certain populations, namely enslaved people and Native Americans, did not seem to suffer from hemiplegia because they did not have the luxury of overthinking and creating more worries for themselves ("The idea of riches never bothers their slumbers"). Please keep in mind that Dr. Still was adamantly against slavery. He and his father joined the anti-slavery Free-Staters. Despite the old language that Dr. Still used in this line, we do not want to undermine the immense suffering endured by both enslaved people and Native Americans and other people of color.

# C

9. **Page 26, "If I should give calomel…"**

    This excerpt is from the *Autobiography of Andrew T. Still*, Chapter XIX, in the section "Calomel and Castor Oil," page 288. Calomel is an inorganic mercury chloride mineral with the formula $Hg_2Cl_2$, also known as mercuric chloride or mercurous chloride. Use of calomel started in the 16th century and continued even until the mid 1900s, despite warnings.

Davis LE. Unregulated potions still cause mercury poisoning. *West J Med*. 2000 Jul;173(1):19. doi: 10.1136/ewjm.173.1.19.

### 10. Page 29, "I think that the cause of croup…"

This line is from *The Philosophy and Mechanical Principles of Osteopathy*, Chapter XVI "Ear-Wax and Its Uses," in the section "An Experiment," page 295.

In Still's time, more infants died from croup than they do today. Fortunately, he had the insight to see how cerumen impaction could irritate the nerves. A visceral reflexive cough can be caused by irritation of the auricular branch of the vagus nerve. In fact, the German anatomist Friedtich Arnold (1803-1890) had observed that irritation to the posterior wall of the external ear canal could elicit a cough in some people. Similarly, other reflexes have also been linked to the auricular branch of the vagus nerve, including a connection between the ear and the heart.

Aaron R. Murray, Lucy Atkinson, Mohd K. Mahadi, Susan A. Deuchars, Jim Deuchars. The strange case of the ear and the heart: The auricular vagus nerve and its influence on cardiac control. *Autonomic Neuroscience*, Volume 199, 2016, pages 48-53.

### 11. Page 31, "More cripples… too thick a diaper…"

The source for this quote could not be found. However, thinking osteopathically, too thick a baby diaper could disrupt the normal development of the articular and ligamentous hip that can have an effect later in life..

### 12. Page 31, "I think consumption begins by…"

Consumption is an old term for tuberculosis (TB). This quote is from *Philosophy and Principles of Osteopathy*, Chapter VI "The Thorax," in the section "The Effects of Consumption," page 109-110. Dr. Still encourages osteopaths to "enter the field of active exploration, and note the causes… Begin at the brain, … Begin at the atlas, follow it with the searchlight of quickened reason, … See what nerve fibers pass through and on to the base and center, and each minute cell, fascia, gland, and blood-vessel of the lungs."

# D

### 13. Page 37, "Bacteria do not cause disease…"

This line is a variation of a line in *The Philosophy and Mechanical Principles of Osteopathy*, Chapter VIII "The Abdomen," from a section entitled "How About Nature?" on pages 163-164. The exact line is as follows:

"I want to impress upon you that all bad sputa, poor lymph, and defective blood are effects only, and a broken link is the cause, and bacteria are only the buzzards formed by the biogen that is in the dead blood itself."

Regarding bacteria, fungi, parasites, microbes, germs, and other "infectious" pathogens, Still also writes, "I do not wish to disprove their existence, but wish to take such witnesses and try to prove that all such abnormal changes have a cause in suspension of arterial or venous blood, or lymph, the excretory systems, or by their nerve-supply being cut off at some important point of the physical work."

In other words, according to Still, infection is not the cause but rather the effect of obstructions and poor circulation.

### 14. Page 40, "Electric shocks in digestion…"

This excerpt is from *The Philosophy and Mechanical Principles of Osteopathy*, Chapter VI "The Thorax," in the section "The Philosophy of Digestion," page 120. Here is more on electricity and digestion from *Osteopathy, Research, and Practice*, in the chapter on Digestion, pages 191-192, paragraph 328:

"Today we know about as little of the process of atomizing food as Adam and Eve did when they ate their first apples. We find fluids of different kinds in the stomach, bowel, pancreas, liver, omentum and peritoneum. We analyze them and find differences in the substances of each division. We name each fluid, talk of chemical action, call this process digestion and stop. We find that fluids are collected in a tank called the receptaculum chyli and from there they are conducted by way of the thoracic duct to the veins, the heart, thence to the lungs and here we drop the subject of digestion. We ask no questions of Edison, Morse or Franklin about the power of electricity to atomize food or to explode compounds while in the stomach. Perhaps an electrician would tell us that the heart is a dynamo, the brain is a storage battery, and the nerves are the wires that conduct the electricity to the stomach and bowels where it atomizes the food. Perhaps Edison would say the stomach and bowels are only vessels to hold the chemical compounds till electricity produces the act of combustion, and that electric combustion is all there is to digestion."

## E

15. **Page 42, "For what purpose… ear-wax?"**

    Still has a whole chapter dedicated to "Ear-Wax and Its Uses" in *The Philosophy and Mechanical Principles of Osteopathy*, Chapter XIV, pages 294-301. From our current understanding, ear wax has multiple purposes, including protecting and cleaning the external ear canal, and maintaining the ear microbiome.

    Hanson, M. and Adams, M. Follow the Wax: The Natural Protection of the Ear Canal and its Biome. *Otolaryngology Clinic N Am*, 56 (2023) 863-867.

16. **Page 44, "The internal mammary…"**

The source of this exact quote could not be found. However, there is a section in *The Philosophy and Mechanical Principles of Osteopathy* Chapter VI - Thorax, dedicated to "The Internal and External Mammary Arteries" on page 131 with the following:

"A confused and suspended circulation, either of the arterial, venous or lymphatic circulation or a disturbance of the nerves of either the arterial, venous or lymphatic circulation of the mammary glands, would be cause sufficient to draw the attention of the osteopathic diagnostician to a very careful investigation of the causes of disease of these glands. He should know that the mammary artery is not oppressed or disturbed by ribs that have been pushed or knocked from their articulation with the sternum or spine, before he would be justified in giving a scientific diagnosis of the cause of tumors of the breast, goitre, diseases of the tonsils, the glands and lymphatics of the neck or breast, the eyes, or the giving way of important functions of any organ, internal or external, of the whole chest. We must remember that the internal mammary is a very long artery, beginning at the first rib and extending to the pelvis. Much good health depends upon its good work, and much bad health and disturbance can reasonably be expected to follow imperfect supply by arterial action or imperfect drainage through the venous and lymphatic vessels."

Regarding the lymphatic and venous drainage, it is easy to understand how blocked plumbing of the mammary vessels could affect the head, neck and thorax.

Digging deeper, let's ask ourselves, how do the internal mammary arteries (IMA) connect with the eyes? Knowing all parts are connected to the whole, we can think about this osteopathically. (Note that the internal mammary artery is an older term for the internal thoracic artery.) Just as the foot can influence the head, so can the IMA affect the eyes. The fulcrum of an issue could potentially be anywhere. The IMA and vertebral arteries arise from the subclavian artery. Any restriction of arterial flow to the subclavian, such as in thoracic outlet syndrome, could have a possible effect on the visual system in more than one way. First, the vertebral arteries supply the primary visual cortex in the occipital lobe. Second, both the anterior and posterior neuro-endocrine-lymphatic points (Chapman's points) of the eye are also supplied by branches of the subclavian artery. Third, the internal and external rotational movements of the various artery segments can affect the blood flow through branches above and below that segment. For there to be optimal flow, all branches of the river of life must flow freely.

## F

**17. Page 50, "Lungs have five lobes…"**

This passage is the entire section on "The Law of Fives" which is in *Philosophy of Osteopathy*, Chapter V "Disease of the Chest," page 59.

**18. Page 53, "The field is already overcrowded with Doctors who…"**

See annotation #4.

## G

**19. Page 61, "I quote no authors but God and experience."**

This is the opening sentence for *The Philosophy and Mechanical Principles of Osteopathy*, Introduction, "My Authorities," Page 9.

# H

### 20. Page 65, "The heart ... does not pull or push..."

The source of this passage could not be found. However, there is growing evidence and understanding that the heart is not a pressure propulsion system. Historically, Ruldolf Steiner (1861–1925), a scientific, literary, and philosophical scholar, spoke to physicians in 1920 about how the blood was "propelled with its own biological momentum." Then, in 1932, a Harvard study led by J.L. Bremer showed that blood circulated in chick embryos in a "self-propelled mode in spiraling streams before the heart was functioning."

Marinelli, Ralph et al. The Heart is Not a Pump: A Refutation of the Pressure Propulsion Premise of Heart Function. *Frontier Perspectives*, (Temple University) Fall-Winter 1995.

The osteopathic profession continues to add to our understanding of the heart's function with *Osteopathy is in the Blood: The Science and Clinical Application of the Rule of the Artery* by Maxwell Fraval, DO (UK) and other contributors (2024). As Dr. Fraval and colleagues emphasize, the heart is a generator, not a pump.

See also the excerpt in Note #14 in which Dr. Still writes, "the heart is a dynamo, the brain is a storage battery..."

### 21. Page 66, "The heart the fountain of life...imparts the attributes of life and knowledge..."

This line is from *Osteopathy, Research, and Practice*, page 182, paragraph 318.

Here is a similar idea from the *Autobiography of Andrew T. Still*, Chapter XXX, in a section on "Who Discovered Osteopathy?" page 417:

"The arteries bring the blood and wash it with the spirit of life. The living arteries from this world. It [the spirit of life] fills all space and forms the clouds."

Research from the HeartMath Institute aligns with Dr. Still's observations. As Rollin McCraty, Ph.D., wrote:

"These changes in electromagnetic, sound pressure, and blood pressure waves produced by cardiac rhythmic activity are "felt" by every cell in the body, further supporting the heart's role as a global internal synchronizing signal."

—The Energetic Heart: Bioelectromagnetic Communication Within and Between People, chapter published in *Clinical Applications of Bioelectromagnetic Medicine*, edited by P. J. Rosch; M. S. Markov. New York: Marcel Dekker, 2004: 541-562.

## 22. Page 69, "I believe all immunities are based on…"

This excerpt is from *The Philosophy and Mechanical Principles of Osteopathy*, Chapter XII "Smallpox," in a section on "Good Nursing," page 287. To give context, here are the few sentences appearing just before this excerpt:

"But, as man's germicidal powers cannot resist the smallpox, he must try to arm himself with an artificial substitute, which I believe we can do and have done with wonderful success in the use of the cantharidin as now reported in hundreds of cases. It creates an infectious fever that is innocent in after-effects, and will hold full possession of the body and defend it from all other infections whilst it has possession, and be a perfect immunity to smallpox at last."

# K

## 23. Page 72, "There are two very large and powerful rivers… the Klondike of life…"

This excerpt is a combination of two passages in Chapter XV on "Convulsions" in *The Philosophy and*

*Mechanical Principles of Osteopathy*, pages 302-303. The first part is from the opening section "Old Systems Unreliable," and the second part is immediately after in the section "Panning for Gold."

The Klondike is a reference to the Klondike River in Canada's Yukon Territory and the Gold Rush of the late 1800s. Here's more about that:

"In the winter of 1897-1898, word spread like wildfire that gold had been discovered along the Klondike River in Canada's Yukon Territory. Men and women from all over the world converged on the area, and two small settlements, Skagway and Dyea (both in Alaska), became competing boomtowns, each claiming it had the easier path to the gold fields. The route of choice for many "stampeders" was the 33-mile-long Chilkoot Trail that began at Dyea and bypassed—so its boosters claimed—the crime of Skagway and the "gridlock" of its White Pass Trail. Some 25,000 to 30,000 people passed through Dyea and traveled the Chilkoot, portions of which were so narrow that sleds and pack animals were almost useless. The worst part of the trail was known as the "Golden Stairs"—1,500 steep steps carved out of ice and snow."

—Banyasz, M.G. Klondike River, Canada. *Archaeology Magazine*, May/June, 2012.

## L

### 24. Page 78, "In death the lymphatics are dark, ..."

This quote is from *Philosophy and Principles of Osteopathy*, Chapter II "Some Substances of the Body, in a section called "Universally Distributed," page 68. The line is referring to how the lymphatics purify the fluids of the blood. The next paragraph starts as follows:

"What we meet with in all diseases is dead blood, stagnant lymph, and albumen in a semi-vital or dead and decomposing condition all through the lymphatics and other parts of the body, brain, lungs, kidneys, liver, and fascia. The whole system is loaded with a confused mass of blood that is mixed with unhealthy substances that should have been kept washed out by lymph."

### 25. Page 81, "According to every method of reasoning…"

This line is from *Osteopathy, Research, and Practice*, Chapter "Organs as Functionaries," page 29, paragraph 50. The exact quote is written with the GREAT I AM in all caps as follows:

"According to every method of reasoning the lung comes in as the GREAT I AM of living blood."

In other words, the breath enlivens the blood with spirit, the breath of life. When we inspire, we breathe in spirit.

### 26. Page 82, "Life in man…region of the heart is his headquarters…"

This excerpt is from *Osteopathy, Research and Practice*, Chapter "Life," in the section "Life in Form," page 513, paragraph 910.

According to research from the HeartMath Institute, the heart's electrical field is about 60 times greater than that of the brain, and the heart's magnetic field is more than 100 times greater than the brain's. There are also more nerve connections from the heart to the brain than the brain to the heart.

# M

### 27. Page 88, "All the processes of earth life must be in perpetual motion…"

This line is from *The Philosophy and Mechanical Principles of Osteopathy (PMPO)*, Chapter X "Fevers", in a section on "Perfection in Nature", page 232.

**Also, on Page 84, "Motion is the first and only evidence of life"**

This line is also from *PMPO*, Chapter XI "Biogen," in a section on "The Origin of Action," pages 249-250. Here is a larger part of that excerpt:

"Then the mind is asked to find the connection between the physical and the spiritual. By Nature you can reason that the powers of life are arranged to suit its system of motion. If life is an individualized personage, as we might express that mysterious something, it must have definite arrangements by which it can be united and act with matter. Then we should acquaint ourselves with the arrangements of those natural connections, the one or many, in all parts of the completed being. As motion is the first and only evidence of life, by this thought we are conducted to the machinery through which life works to accomplish the result as witnessed in 'motion'."

Note that, R. Paul Lee, D.O., referenced this passage in his article "Spirituality in Osteopathic Medicine," in the Winter, 2000, *The American Academy of Osteopathy Journal*, Vol 31.

28. **Page 88, "We must remember that the internal mammary…"**

This excerpt is from *The Philosophy and Mechanical Principles of Osteopathy*, Chapter VI, "The Thorax," in a section on "Rheumatism," page 131. The internal mammary artery (IMA), also known as the internal thoracic artery, arises from the subclavian artery and supplies the anterior chest wall and breasts, including the mediastinum, thymus, sternum, and ribs. Once the IMA passes through the diaphragm, it has anastomoses with the abdominal and pelvic arteries, from the celiac artery to the external iliac artery.

**29. Page 114, "No breast should become caked…"**

This line refers to the treatment of mastitis and is from *The Philosophy and Mechanical Principles of Osteopathy*, Chapter XVI "Obstetrics", in a section on "Treatment of the Breast," page 318.

# P

**30. Page 117, "My object is to make the Osteopath a philosopher…"**

Dr. Still emphasized teaching concepts to learn the art of medicine. Although the source of this exact line could not be found, Still often spoke of osteopaths as philosophers, as exemplified in the following excerpt from *Autobiography of Andrew T. Still*, pages 404-405:

"I would advise you to take up the philosophy, and learn all you can about it, for you know the questions will come. I am satisfied and pleased to have the people ask questions and receive all the answers they can get. And after I have answered all I can through the papers or with my own mouth, I cannot even answer a moiety of them. To answer all the questions that are suggested by a human thigh-bone would open and close an eternity. Therefore you must not expect me to answer all of them. Neither must you expect this school to do that for you. You can get enough demonstrations to put you on the track to become a self-generating philosopher. It is as full of suggestions as the rising of the sun, the opening of the mouths of vegetation when the evening shades appear-moon-flowers, night-flowers, and all others opening their mouths to draw life from the bosom of God. The most sublime thought I ever had in my life is concerning the machinery, and the works as I found them in the human construction, faithfully executing all of the known duties and the beauties of life."

### 31. Page 119, "Biogen is the lives of the two in unified action…"

This excerpt is from *The Philosophy and Mechanical Principles of Osteopathy (PMPO)*, Chapter XI "Biogen," in a section "Forces Combined," page 251. Here are some other lines from that paragraph:

"Thus endowed, two beings or worlds, when in contact, give wisdom and force to work out greater problems than either could accomplish alone. … The celestial worlds of space or ether-life give forms wisely constructed in exchange for the use of the material substances. Reciprocity through the governments of the celestial and terrestrial worlds is ever the same, and human life, in form and motion, is the result of conception by the terrestrial mother from the celestial father. Thus we have a union of mind, matter, and life, or man."

Along these lines, Dr. Still also wrote about "Man is Triune" on pages in the Introduction to *PMPO* on pages 16-17. Here is a brief excerpt:

"…and after all our explorations, we have to decide that man is triune when complete.

First, there is the material body; second, the spiritual being; third, a being of mind which is far superior to all vital motions and material forms, whose duty is to wisely manage this great engine of life."

### 32. Page 121, "Prophecy is what can be seen by a cloudless mind…"

This line is from *The Philosophy and Mechanical Principles of Osteopathy (PMPO)*, Chapter XXVII, subheading "Prophecy," page 390.

Related to the section on Prophecy, is the "Intuitive Mind" in Chapter XXIX on page 407 of *PMPO*, in which Dr. A.T. Still tells a story of how his father, who was both a physician and minister, was a "sensitive man and had an intuitive mind." The senior Dr. Still intuitively knew just when he was needed for emergencies, even traveling fifty to seventy miles based on his "intuitive mind" alone.

Dr. Still also wrote about intuition in a section entitled "Intuitive Consciousness," which was in the November, 1898, *Journal of Osteopathy,* Vol 5, No 6. Here is a copy of that passage:

"By following a study with practical training, a person becomes acquainted with the principles to such fullness that he can do good work in all parts, and feels no farther effort will be required. He does his work well and feels so, because of his being master of his trade by practical experience and close observation to the study while an apprentice. Another person of his apprentice class who never lost an hour, cannot do as good work, and lives a life of confused labor, but stands about par in all other branches. The first man has obtained from study something that the second man has not. The first drives through all kinds of difficult problems with ease, while number two is almost a failure in all places. Why the difference? Perhaps number one has worked for and obtained intuitive consciousness, or made all subjects to his mind beings of life, that live under laws made for their being. He who succeeds must study the law of all pursuits or trades. To observe and obey is the only way to succeed; he does succeed by obedience to such laws until mind and body becomes equally sensitive to the fact that man must feel that he is right before he can be successful.

By the law of knowledge and intuition all persons do succeed. Thus we should not be satisfied to know that we are right, but feel so, and act with energy to suit, and our successes will grow with time. We must feel an interest in all we do or we will always eat at the table of disappointment.

It may be possible that we do not think often enough of man's dual nature, and that his body is under his mind, and obeys its orders all the time. By long service under the mind the body becomes saturated so thoroughly with the telegraphy of thought that it feels premonitions of an order to execute some duty before the order is given; perhaps from the fact that the body is full of the essence of mind and its action. I will drop this thought and say, that the above is only an immature suggestion. I believe the greatest blessing we can obtain is to have sensation in union and action with mind and body if we would succeed."

# Q

### 33. Page 127-128, Chapter Q, "Questions for Osteopaths"

This entire chapter was taken from *The Philosophy and Mechanical Principles of Osteopathy*, in the chapter "Biogen," subheading "The Appearance of Œdema, pages 265-268. Note there were a handful of word and conjugation changes, as well as the possibly accidental omission of one question. Here are the original questions:

- "Œdema is one word that appears at the first showing of life and death in animal forms. ...

- Has Nature furnished man with powers to make his bones and give them the necessary form?

- Does a section in Nature's law provide fastenings to hold these to one another?

- How will this body move, and where and how is the force applied?

- Where and how is this force obtained?

- How is it generated and supplied to these parts of motion?

- What makes these muscles, ligaments, nerves, veins, and arteries?

- Are they self-forming, or has Nature prepared

machinery to make them?

- Does animal life contain knowledge and force for the construction of all the parts of man?
- Can it run the machine after it has finished it?
- By what power does it move?
- Is there a blood-vessel running to every part of this body to supply all these demands?
- If it has a battery of force, where is it?
- What does it use for force
- Is it electricity? If so, how does it collect and use this substance? How does it convey its powers?
- How does man keep warm without a fire?
- How does he build and lose flesh all the time?
- Where and how is the supply made and delivered to proper places?
- How is it applied and what holds it to its place when adjusted?
- What makes it build the house of life?
- Do demand and supply govern the work? If not, what does? [Note this line was omitted.]
- Are the laws of animal life sufficient to do all this work of building and repairing wastes and keeping it in running condition?
- If they are, what can man do or suggest to help them?
- Is this machine capable of being run fast or slow if need be?
- Does man have in him some kind of chemical laboratory that can turn out such products as he needs to fill all his physical demands?
- If by heat, exercise, or any other cause he gets warm, can that chemistry cool him to normal?

- If too cold, can it warm him? Can it adjust him to heat and cold?
- If so, how is it done? Is the law of life and longevity fully vindicated in man's make-up?"

# S

### 34. Page 138, "We are warranted to conclude that Nature…"

This passage is from *Autobiography of Andrew T. Still*, Chapter XVI, "The Solvent Powers of Life," pages 251-252. Another line from this same section provides more detail:

"We would renovate first by lymph, giving it time to do its work of atomizing all crudities first. Then we can expect to see the effect of growing processes as a natural result."

# T

### 35. Page 144, "We often speak of Truth. A truth is the complete work of Nature,…"

This excerpt is from *The Philosophy and Mechanical Principles of Osteopathy*, page 15, in a section entitled, "Truth Is Truth." Here are the lines leading up to the excerpt:

"But no one truth is greater than any other truth. Each has a sphere of usefulness peculiar to itself. Thus we should treat with respect and reverence all truths, great and small."

# U

### 36. Page 149, "In urinalysis you are told, …"

This passage is from *The Philosophy and Mechanical Principles of Osteopathy*, Chapter VIII "The Abdomen," in the section "The Thoracic Duct," page 151. Here is another sentence leading up to this line:

"Is it not reasonable to suppose that a ligation of the thoracic duct at the diaphragm would retain this chyle until it would be diseased by age and fermentation, and be thrown off into the substances of other organs of the abdomen, setting up new growths, such as enlargement of the uterus, ovaries, kidneys, liver, spleen, pancreas, omentum, lymphatics, cellular membranes, and all that is known as flesh and blood below the diaphragm?"

# W

37. **Page 152, "'Wind' and wisdom never blend."**

    This line is from *Autobiography of Andrew T. Still*, page 166. Here's more from that paragraph:

    "Another kind of danger stands in the background, a too-much-talk man; he talks continually and thinks but little. "Wind" and wisdom never blend."

38. **Page 153, "The one is the upper stomach…"**

    This excerpt is from *Philosophy of Osteopathy*, Chapter XVII "Obstetrics," section on "Overloading" and "Similarity of Stomach and Womb," pages 141-142.

# Index

**A...pages 13-17**
    adjuncts: pg 16
    adjustment: pp 15, 21-22, 32, 51, 62, 69, 83-84, 91-93, 97-99, 101, 109, 113, 114, 128, 129, 132, 148-149
        adjust our telescopes: pg 62
        bony adjustment: pp 15, 21-22, 149
        adjustment, disease or remedies: pp 33, 36, 93, 114, 132
        adjust the machinery: pp 32, 91-92, 98-99, 101, 109
        Nature's plans and specifications: pp 83-84, 97-99, 101
        precision, not too much or too little: pp 15, 69, 109, 113
        and reason: pg 148
        Self-adjusting: pp 51, 159
        snapping and popping: pp 21-22
    advice: pp 16, 132
    age, ages: pp 13, 17, 34, 77, 90, 94, 137, 140, 145, 148
    ambition: pg 15
    anatomy, anatomies, anatomist: pp 13-17, 68, 75, 109, 154
    antidote: pg 13
    ape: pg 16
    architect, architecture: pp 13, 48, 57, 97, 132, 148
    artery, arteries, arterial: pp 13-17, 20-23, 46, 52, 62, 72, 77, 88, 96, 104, 127
        internal mammary artery: pp 166, 172

assisted: pp 13, 14
asthma, asthmatic: pp 14, 16
atlas: pp 17, 143
atom: pp 13, 22, 34, 43, 59-60, 78, 89-90, 121, 151, 154
automobile: pg 15

## B...pages 18-25

babe: pg 22
bed-wetting: pg 46
begin(s), beginning: pp 14, 17, 21, 25-26, 29, 31, 35, 43, 54, 58, 67, 88, 90, 94-95, 113, 124, 143, 145, 152
believe, belief: pp 21, 29, 31, 44, 55, 58, 60, 69, 77, 79, 83, 93, 114, 122, 150
biogen: pp 89, 119-120
bladder: pg 23
blood, blood stream: pp 14-15, 18-25, 33-35, 38, 45, 47-48, 53-54, 60, 62, 64, 66, 71, 77, 79-82, 85, 89, 99, 101, 103, 106, 113-114, 116, 121, 128, 137, 139, 146
boat(s): pp 20, 25, 65, 146
body, bodies: pp 14, 18, 19-26, 28, 31-39, 41, 43-45, 47-53, 55-58, 60-63, 65-66, 69, 72, 75, 77-79, 81-82, 86, 89-91, 93-94, 98, 103-104, 110, 112, 114, 117-120, 122-124, 127-128, 131-132, 136, 140, 145, 148-150, 153, 158-159, 161-162, 169-171, 174-177
boiler: pg 20
bone, bones: pp 17, 19, 21-22, 30, 52, 58, 64, 76, 99, 109-110, 113, 125, 127, 137-138, 159-160, 173, 176
boots: pp 18, 68
borrow(s): pp 24, 65
bowel(s): pp 50, 54, 59, 61, 121, 124, 134, 165
brace: pg 22
brains: pp 15, 18, 22-25, 34, 42-43, 46, 49, 52, 55, 64, 66-67, 76-78, 82-83, 85, 88, 103, 136, 153-154
brawn: pg 18
Bright's Disease, bright: pp 21, 149
brother, brotherhood: pp 18-20, 23, 109, 136
building: pp 21, 25, 48, 92, 97, 128, 148, 168
business: pp 16, 19, 28, 45, 51, 54-55, 73, 80, 110, 146, 158
button: pg 19

## C...pages 26-32

calomel: pp 26, 158
cancer: pg 26
cat: pp 27, 92
cause: pp 14, 16, 26-32, 34, 37, 39, 43, 45, 54, 56-57, 64, 77, 79, 82, 85, 89, 106, 112, 117-118, 121-122, 124-126, 129, 131, 133-134, 137-138, 140, 143, 145, 148-149, 153, 162-164, 166, 175, 177
cerebrospinal fluid, cerebro-spinal fluid, CSF: pp 31, 43, 52, 104
cerumen, earwax, ear wax, ear-wax: pp 29, 42-43, 100, 163, 165
channel(s): pp 13, 20, 25, 27, 29, 31, 34, 39-40, 103, 145
chemical(s): pp 24, 28, 31-33, 40, 59, 61, 85, 92, 94, 101, 120, 129, 138, 165, 177
chemistry, chemistries: pp 24, 31-32, 87, 129, 177
cinder(s): pg 50
circulation: pp 29, 65, 79, 82, 164, 166
clairvoyance: pg 32
climb: pp 28, 30
college(s): pg 30
comprehension: pg 29
condition(s): pp 27, 29-30, 39, 43, 60, 64, 66, 70, 77, 84, 88, 92, 95, 110, 123-124, 130, 138, 147, 162
confidence: pp 28, 31, 57, 73, 126, 138
conjecture(s): pg 28
constipation: pg 30
construct, construction: pp 14, 22-23, 25, 29, 40-41, 48, 59, 68, 76, 79, 83, 90-91, 95-96, 114, 118-119, 123, 127, 138, 154, 173-174, 177
consumption: pp 31, 163-164
contagious, contagion: pp 29, 69
coon: pg 28
corpuscle(s): pp 20, 27, 32, 101, 138
courage: pp 18, 28, 63
cripple(s): pp 31, 65, 163
cure: pp 26, 33, 36-37, 43, 47, 59, 64, 93, 101, 105-106, 111, 113, 118, 126

## D...pages 33-40

death: pp 33-35, 37-38, 43, 48, 54-55, 61, 76, 78, 84, 86, 90, 99, 114, 120, 144, 148, 170, 176
decomposition: pp 38, 118, 125
defect(s), defective: pp 35-36, 97, 164
Deity: pp 36, 62, 93

demand(s): pp 17, 34, 37, 53, 58, 97, 100, 103-104, 124, 128-129, 138, 177
destination: pp 34, 77
develop(s), development: pp 26, 33, 38-40, 51, 62, 84, 99, 102, 159, 163
diaphragm pp 20, 35, 39, 52, 72, 149
digestion, indigestion: pp 34, 38-40, 43, 45, 59-60
discover, discovery: pp 34, 44, 100, 109
disease(s): pp 13-14, 21, 26-27, 29, 31, 33-41, 43, 45, 51, 54, 61, 64, 66-67, 73, 77, 79, 85, 89, 93, 98, 106, 108, 110, 115-116, 118, 120, 122-124, 134, 136, 139, 146, 149-150, 164, 166-167, 170, 179
dissection: pp 26, 37, 109
Divine: pp 28, 51, 57, 107, 113, 137
doctor: pp 15, 23, 33, 36-37, 49, 53-54, 59, 62, 71, 78-79, 81-82, 93-94, 98, 101, 106, 108, 123-125, 130-132, 137, 150
dorsal: pp 33, 126
drainage: pp 36, 161
drug(s): pp 19, 26, 33-37, 53, 61-62, 81, 88, 93, 96, 101, 108, 121, 139
drunkenness: pg 38

## E...pages 41-46

ear(s): pp 36, 45, 67
ear wax (see cerumen): pp 29, 42-43, 100, 163, 165
earth: pp 39-40, 44, 74, 84, 88, 119, 121-122, 146, 171
eat: pp 44, 46-47, 50, 52, 63, 73, 120, 175
edema: pp 43, 176
ego: pg 44
electric: pp 34, 40, 43, 51, 88, 111, 159, 164-165
Electrician: pp 43, 111, 165, 177
electricity: pp 41, 45-46, 49, 54, 58, 66, 128, 149, 153, 159, 164-165
    pectoral electricity: pg 67
electro-magnet, electromagnetic: pp 17, 85, 131, 169
element(s): pp 31-32, 43, 95, 97, 99, 101, 118
emotion: pg 95
engine: pp 17, 35, 41, 44-45, 76, 84, 92, 130, 134, 148, 174
engineer(s), engineering: pp 41, 44-46, 91, 97-98, 102, 145, 161
enuresis, nocturnal enuresis (see bed-wetting): pg 46
enterprise: pg 44
environment: pp 26, 123
equilibrium: pg 45
existence: pp 42, 112, 164

eye(s): pp 24, 26, 36, 44-47, 55, 67, 72, 77, 81, 97, 103, 108, 125, 130, 135-136, 139, 147, 166-167

## F...pages 47-56

fact(s): pp 25, 52, 100, 126, 131, 135, 147-148
failure: pp 23, 27, 35, 38, 54, 58, 73, 81, 104, 117, 121, 135, 152, 175
faith, faithfulness: pp 23, 49, 54, 61, 76, 79, 100-101, 107, 114
Fascia: pp 35, 46, 48, 54-55, 76, 85
father: pp 14, 49, 118, 147, 162, 174
feet, foot: pp 49, 68, 74, 94, 126, 135, 167
female: pp 51, 55
fermentation, fermenation [sic]: pp 38, 56, 85-86, 118, 128, 179
fever: pp 47-51, 53, 65, 86, 143, 153, 159, 169, 171
field: pp 43, 53, 67, 69, 115, 123, 131, 144, 152, 154, 160, 164, 167, 170-171
fight: pp 13, 48, 75, 107, 139
finders and fixers, find and fix, find it fix it: pp 50, 53, 149
fire, afire: pp 26, 30, 49-51, 53, 80, 128, 143, 153
fireman: pg 50
fit(s), seizure(s): pp 51-52
five: pp 50, 63, 95, 137, 167
fluid(s): pp 20, 23, 27, 31, 34-35, 37, 39, 42-43, 47, 49, 51-52, 54-55, 57, 61, 65-66, 72, 83, 85, 89, 100, 114, 120, 130, 134, 137-139, 165, 170
   amniotic fluids: pg 64
   boiling of the fluids: pg 56
   finer fluids: pg 83
   fluids of life: pp 27, 89
   gas, fluids, or solids: pp 34, 42, 47, 51, 61, 66, 120, 137-138
   monthly fluids: pg 55
   red or black fluid: pg 20
   stagnation of fluids: pp 66, 130, 137
   union of fluids: pg 35
framework: pp 17, 55, 69
free: pp 38, 82, 104, 119, 139
freedom: pp 47, 61
food(s): pp 23, 35, 40, 42, 47, 49-52, 59, 98, 123, 126, 144, 159, 165
force(s): pp 15, 19, 24, 29, 37, 41, 43, 53-54, 65, 69, 71, 77-78, 82, 84, 86, 89, 91-92, 95, 98, 104, 111-112, 116, 119-120, 127-128, 131, 135-136, 138-139, 153, 159, 174, 176-177
foundation: pp 47-48, 50, 52, 86, 140, 158
friction: pp 45, 51, 58
fuel: pg 49

fundamental: pp 14, 37, 56, 146
furnace: pp 47, 49

## G...pages 57-61

ganglia: pg 104
ganglion, superior cervical: pg 59
germ(s), germicide, germicidal: pp 29-32, 60-61, 90, 120, 154, 164, 169
God, He, His, Him: pp 13, 19, 21, 28, 34, 42, 49, 57-59, 60-61, 68, 73, 88, 93, 96, 101, 103, 107-108, 112, 118, 121, 131-132, 135, 142-143, 150-151, 153, 158-159, 167, 173
govern: pp 19, 23, 37, 39, 58, 77, 81, 95, 101, 106, 119, 140, 153, 177
governing: pp 41, 58, 83, 114
government: pp 39, 174
Great I Am: pp 81, 171
growth(s): pp 26, 32, 57-58, 119
guess, guessing: pp 58-59, 142, 147
guide: pp 58, 108

## H...pages 62-67

habit: pp 62, 145
habitation: pg 23
hand: pp 17, 29, 64, 106-107, 109, 113, 117, 121
    hand in hand: pg 107, 111, 117
    hand and the head: pp 64, 121
    Nature's hand: pg 29
    work hand: pg 151
happy: pp 63, 94
harmony: pp 19, 21, 62, 64, 99
hay: pp 29, 63
head: pp 27-28, 44, 46, 57-58, 64, 68-69, 71, 78, 100, 109, 117, 121, 131, 146
    bathe your heads: pp 28, 57
    hand in head: pp 64, 121
headache: pg 64
headquarters: pg 82
health: pp 14, 19, 25, 28, 33, 35-36, 39, 43-44, 47, 55, 57-59, 62-67, 72, 75, 78, 81, 84-85, 88, 93, 101, 108-109, 111, 116, 123, 132, 136, 144, 154, 166, 171
heart: pp 13, 20, 25, 29, 44, 49, 53, 60, 62-67, 82, 85, 88, 94, 103, 116, 141, 159, 163, 165, 168-169, 171

heat: pp 19, 24, 40, 47, 50-51, 59, 65, 91, 102, 129, 132, 148, 159, 177-178
heaven: pp 15, 64, 94, 122
hemiplegia: pp 63, 162
hemorrhage: pp 62, 64
homeopathy: pg 62
hope: pp 44, 66, 73, 101, 125, 132, 140, 147
horn(s): pg 63
hurting, hurt: pp 64, 118
hypermobility: pg 66
hypodermic (needle): pg 64

## I...pages 68-70
ignorance: pp 14, 48, 53, 68-70, 72, 82, 88, 90, 117, 139, 145, 147
image: pg 69
imitation(s), imitator: pp 41, 68-69, 96, 123, 125
immune, immunities: pp 60, 69, 82
Infinite: pp 17, 23, 54, 62, 69, 132, 138
inquiry: pp 69, 106
Intelligence: pp 24, 59-61, 68, 81, 83, 93, 107, 126, 132, 127, 148
Irrigate, irrigation: pp 43, 69
Irritation(s), irritate: pp 46, 68, 120, 134, 138, 144, 152, 159, 163

## K...pages 71-74
Kansas: pg 71
kidney: pg 71
king: pp 14, 62, 71
Klondike: pp 72, 85, 169-170
knife: pp 32, 57, 70-73, 88, 99, 115, 123, 143
know, knowing: pp 13, 16, 17, 19-21, 24-25, 27-28, 30, 33, 42-45, 47-49, 51, 53-55, 57-58, 65-66, 68, 71, 73, 76, 78, 80-81, 85, 89, 92, 95-100, 102-103, 107-109, 112, 114, 116-117, 122, 124, 130, 136, 142, 144-146, 148-149, 152-154, 158, 160, 162, 165-166, 168, 170, 172-173, 175, 177, 179
knowledge: pp 13-15, 17, 24, 29-30, 33, 37, 41, 68, 71-74, 78-81, 101, 104, 110-111, 114, 117, 119, 124, 125, 127, 138, 145, 154, 168, 175, 177
    knowledge of cause and effect: pp 138, 145
    knowledge by 'littles': pg 79
    tree of knowledge: pp 72, 74

## L...pages 75-86

laborers: pp 19, 76
large: pp 45, 52, 75, 87, 109
    larger circle: pg 71
large eyes: pg 45
two large rivers: pg 72
law(s) of life, laws that govern life, Nature's laws: pp 31, 39, 73, 75-80, 84, 99-102, 107, 111, 117, 127, 129, 140, 143, 158, 167, 175-178
    law of cause and change in union: pg 31
    law of the free circulation of blood: pg 82
    laws of creation: pg 122
    law of death: pg 84
    law of ejection: pg 153
    law of fermentation: pp 118, 125
    laws governing the engine: pg 41
    laws governing the growth of vegetation: pg 58
    laws of gravitation: pg 65
    laws of health: pg 65
    His law: pp 27, 93
    laws of the Infinite: pg 69
    law of intelligence: pg 81
    laws of union in Nature (chemistry): pg 31
    nutrient law: pp 46, 82
    laws of Osteopathy (not framed by human hands): pp 108-109
    penal law of death: pg 35
    physical laws: pp 13, 75
    Law of possession: pg 69
    laws of reason: pp 124, 130
    laws of the universe: pg 79
Leavings of the medical world: pp 80, 85, 147
legacy: pp 76, 83
lengthen a man's life: pg 78
lever: pp 22, 76
liberty: pg 77
light: pp 17, 21, 44, 67, 80, 92, 108, 117, 124, 135, 144, 164
    lighthouse: pg 108
    lightning: pg 44
    searchlights: pp 67, 117, 124, 144, 164
    sunlight: pg 135
limb(s): pp 43, 65-66, 71-72, 81, 113
liver: pp 37-38, 50, 75, 77, 136, 153

living blood: pp 20, 60, 81
Living God: pp 81, 147
living tree: pg 75
locomotor ataxia: pg 82
longevity: pp 83, 125, 129
lowest animated being: pg 83
lung(s): pp 14, 22-23, 29, 50, 54, 60-61, 77, 79-81, 85, 88, 116, 141, 159, 164-165, 167, 171
lymph, lymphatics: pp 24, 26, 37, 50, 60, 76-78, 80, 83, 85-86, 100, 124, 144-145, 161-162, 164, 166-167, 170-171, 179

**M...pages 87-96**

machine, machinery: pp 14, 30, 32, 35, 47, 52, 57, 59, 76-77, 88, 91, 95, 98-101, 109, 116, 125, 127-129, 144, 146, 151, 172-173, 177
mammary, internal: pp 44, 88, 96, 166, 172
material: pp 24, 35, 40, 59, 79, 83, 89-90, 99, 101-102, 119-120, 127, 135, 153
mathematician: pg 87
matter: pp 29, 43, 60, 78, 89, 172, 174
    life and matter: pp 39, 78, 86, 89-90, 119
    matter in motion: pp 90-91, 99
    mind, matter, and life or man: pp 89-91, 119
mental: pp 17, 32, 37, 56, 67, 79, 80, 82, 87-88, 94-95, 144
methods: pp 39, 53, 60, 67, 71, 81, 88, 109, 113, 115, 120, 134, 145, 153, 171
million(s): pp 34, 87, 154
mites of life to the monsters of the land: pg 87
motion: pp 13, 15, 17, 24, 30, 40-41, 50, 66, 84, 88-92, 95, 99, 108, 114, 117-119, 122, 124, 127, 148, 158-159, 171-172, 174, 176
move, moving: pp 16, 20, 27-28, 48, 51, 53, 64, 76, 78, 82, 86, 89, 99, 103-104, 109, 119, 127-128, 130, 140, 160, 167, 176-177
mule(s): pp 70, 87

**N...pages 97-105**

narcotic: pg 98
neck: pp 17, 31, 102-103, 118, 166
nerve: pp 13, 23, 45, 54, 59, 71, 80, 97, 103-104, 107, 116, 139, 144, 153, 159, 161, 163-166, 171, 176
nervous: pp 45, 82, 102
normal: pp 15, 17, 21, 26-27, 30, 39, 57, 88, 92, 97-98, 113, 123, 143, 149

nourish, nourished: pp 42, 97, 103
nourishment: pp 13, 52, 59, 84, 98, 152
nutrition: pp 25, 30, 42, 50, 54, 66, 97, 104, 162

## O...pages 106-115

obstetrics: pp 113, 173, 179
obstruction: pp 15, 17, 57, 62, 99, 104, 106, 109, 111, 131
omentum: pp 79, 165, 179
opposing force: pg 112
organ(s): pp 23, 35, 38, 46, 48, 53, 64, 66, 73, 79, 81, 83, 91, 96, 109, 111, 114-117, 123, 134, 145
Osteopath: pp 13, 16, 26, 28, 36, 41, 43, 51, 54, 56, 71-72, 80, 82, 85, 91, 99, 101, 105-106, 108-109, 111, 113-114, 117, 120, 122-124, 136-137, 158-176, 178-179
Osteopathic: pp 15, 78, 99, 110, 137, 140, 146

## P...pages 116-126

pain: pp 27, 37, 47, 58, 64, 98, 112, 118, 126
pancreas: pp 165, 179
parrots: pg 124
patient: pp 16, 26, 53, 56, 59, 64-66, 73, 80-81, 93, 96, 101, 103, 106, 112-113, 115, 118, 120, 123, 133, 150
pelvis: pp 64, 88, 113, 121, 124, 134, 145, 166
perfect, perfection: pp 22, 33, 36, 45, 47, 49, 51, 58, 62, 65, 67-68, 76, 81-82, 94, 97, 103-104, 109, 116-117, 120-122, 138, 166, 169, 171
 imperfect, imperfection: pp 27, 48, 78, 90-91, 133, 166
person: pp 42, 46, 66, 81, 102, 109, 172, 175
philosopher: pp 81-82, 102, 117, 119, 123-125, 148, 173
philosophy: pp 38, 69, 114, 117, 119-120, 134, 145, 148
physician: pp 15, 52, 53, 98, 110, 112, 118, 126, 137, 146, 160, 168, 174
physiology: pp 43, 58, 68
piles: pp 103, 121
pills: pp 26, 58, 68, 121, 123, 137
plant, planted: pp 22, 39, 90, 119, 132
poison, poisonous: pp 13, 29, 37, 50, 52, 61, 66, 68, 94, 117-118, 120-125, 134, 139
polyps: pg 116

power: pp 21, 23, 29, 35-36, 43-44, 47-48, 51-52, 60, 63, 69, 72-73, 76, 84, 90-91, 94-95, 103-104, 110, 116, 118-119, 121, 124-125, 127-128, 133, 136-139, 144, 146, 148, 154, 159, 165, 169, 172, 176-178
    powerful acid: pg 73
    brain or nerve power: pp 21, 103, 121, 136
    keen power: pg 23
    healing power: pg 110
    powers of life (and death): pp 29, 35, 52, 60, 63, 84, 91
    machinery power: pp 47, 52, 76, 116, 127, 144
    power of mental gratitude: pg 94
    mental/ mind power: pp 95, 113
    powerful microscope: pp 36, 43
    power to move: pg 119
    Nature's power: pp 118, 138-139
    no power: pg 125
    nutrition and power: pg 104
    own power: pg 51
    reasoning powers: pp 90, 103, 148, 153-154
    powerful remedy: pg 48
    powerful rivers: pg 72
    solvent powers: pp 137-138
    power of thunder and lightening: pg 44
    powerful in truth: pg 47
pray, prayer: pp 28, 57, 68, 116
principles: pp 14, 22, 37, 50, 57, 76, 81, 99, 101, 105, 115, 117-120, 122-123, 148
prize: pg 122
professional: pp 96, 123
progress: pp 68, 107, 111, 117-118, 136
prophecy: pp 121, 174
prostate: pg 116
prostration: pg 125
protective: pg 120
    self-protecting: pg 99
public: pp 18, 88, 126
puke, purge, purgative: pp 94, 107

## Q (Questions)...pages 127-129

## R...pages 130-133

relapse: pg 130
remedy: pp 15, 33, 48, 101, 106, 122, 132, 135
remember: pp 17, 23, 37, 54, 64, 72, 80, 88, 99, 106, 131, 137
renovate: pp 104, 131, 178
respect: pp 26, 44, 51, 55, 59, 77, 101, 132, 137, 142, 154, 178
results: pp 14, 24, 26, 29, 58, 64, 66, 87, 91, 100-101, 111, 114, 119, 132, 136, 142, 147
rib: pp 88, 133, 136, 166, 172
road: pp 31, 64, 66-67, 84, 94, 110, 131-132, 144
rule of the artery: pp 13, 21
ruts of allopathy: pg 49

## S...pages 134-141

sac: pp 64, 134
sacred: pp 35, 57, 84, 110, 139, 145
sacro-iliac joint: pp 15-16
satisfaction: pg 136
school: pp 32, 59, 61, 80, 97, 101-102, 104-106, 123-124, 136-137, 139, 160, 173
science: pp 36, 77, 93, 107, 109-110, 112, 115, 117, 136-137, 139-140, 142, 147, 161, 168
sense(s): pp 50, 63, 95, 100, 137
    good or common sense: pp 63, 87, 126
shocks: pp 34, 40, 64, 139, 164
sickness: pp 58, 71, 86, 88, 94, 118, 134, 137, 142
skill: pp 15, 26, 42, 71, 82, 90-91, 95, 98, 111, 139, 154
slaughter-pens: pg 138
solvent: pp 132, 137-138, 161, 178
spine: pp 16, 46, 51, 66, 73, 113, 136-137, 144, 146, 166
Spirit, spiritual: pp 14, 119, 135, 168, 171-172, 174
squirrel: pp 30, 140
stomach: pp 134
structure: pp 37, 92, 110, 123, 135, 137, 140, 146, 149
study: pp 15, 17, 34, 51, 55, 69, 83, 87, 91, 101, 118, 137, 139-140, 160, 168, 175
stupidity: pp 18, 53, 136, 138
substances: pp 14, 22, 25, 29, 31, 39-40, 42, 54, 76, 86, 128, 138, 153
    finely prepared substance: pg 78
    poisonous substances: pg 120
    substance known as life, living substance: pp 81-82, 86, 136, 148

success, successful: pp 15, 18, 67-68, 72-74, 79, 85, 94, 99-100, 102, 117, 124, 135-136, 138, 140, 145, 160, 169, 175
sunlight: pg 135
surgery: pp 26, 72, 110, 123, 135, 137, 140
symphysis: pp 64, 107, 138
symptoms: pp 26, 139

## T...pages 142-148

talk(s): pp 18, 44, 46, 102, 136, 146, 148
temperature: pp 49, 148, 159
theory: pp 32, 138
thinker: pp 142, 146-147
thought: pp 16, 19, 25-26, 36, 49, 54-55, 65-67, 76, 85, 91, 98, 101, 121, 135, 138, 143, 146-147, 162, 172-173, 176
time: pp 18, 21, 28-30, 37, 45-48, 54, 65, 71, 73-74, 79-80, 87, 97, 102-104, 106, 112, 117, 123, 128, 137-138, 140, 143, 146-147, 149, 151, 163, 171, 175-178
timidity: pg 145
tinker: pg 146
tonsil(s): pp 36, 46, 143, 146, 166
tracks of God: pg 143
tradition: pp 143, 145, 147
tree: pp 22, 28, 30, 75, 114, 119, 132, 136
    circulatory tree: pg 65
    coon in tree: pg 28
    tree of knowledge/life: pp 72, 74, 147
    squirrel in the tree: pp 30, 140
truth: pp 25, 44, 46-47, 58, 63, 87-88, 93, 99, 109, 115, 130-132, 135, 140, 142-144, 146-148, 178
tumefaction, tumefying: pp 29, 143, 145
tumor: pp 14, 21, 46, 116, 145, 166
typhus: pp 143, 159

## U...page 149

unity: pg 149
Universe: pp 81, 82, 95
    Grand Architect of the Universe: pg 13
    laws of the Universe: pg 79
    Mind of the Universe: pg 86
    miniature Universe within man: pg 149
    principles govern the Universe: pp 101, 105
    temperature regulates the motion: pg 148

urinalysis: pp 149, 178
uses: pp 20, 23, 24, 41, 43-44, 49-50, 55, 61, 71, 78, 83, 95, 120, 139, 149, 163, 165

**V...pages 150-151**
veins: pp 13-14, 20, 24, 52, 62, 72, 127, 150, 165, 176
   venous: pp 26, 38, 46, 60, 150, 164, 166
venereal: pg 150
visions: pp 25, 35, 49-50, 55, 61, 81, 84, 151

**W...pages 152-154**
war: pp 146, 153
water: pp 13-14, 23-24, 110, 143, 151
   cloud of water: pg 153
   water ducts in childbirth: pg 23
   waters of the Dead Sea, veins: pp 25, 150
   goose on water: pg 122
   living water, waters of life: pp 55, 76, 82
   water from the lymphatics: pp 49, 124
   mechanics of water: pg 111
   pure waters of reason: pg 130
   sulphuric acid in water: pg 13
weigh, weight, weighed: pp 23, 153
willing: pp 71, 79, 99, 102, 152
wind: pp 58, 83, 131, 152-153, 179
wisdom: pp 19, 35, 58, 60, 78-80, 90, 96, 103, 119-120, 147, 150, 152, 154, 174, 179
wise: pp 17, 20, 29, 36-37, 42, 51, 55, 59, 63, 67, 77, 84-85, 95, 102-104, 115
wheels: pp 34, 92, 154
woman: pp 37, 55, 73, 140, 152
womb: pp 55, 138, 152, 179
wonder: pp 44, 49, 67, 92, 110, 153
worship: pp 60, 154
works: pp 36, 60, 62, 76, 87, 91, 98, 104, 121, 135, 153, 165, 166
wound: pp 78, 83, 114, 152

*Let your eyes be a microscope of the greatest known power. Let your mind penetrate to the remotest period of thought by the telescope of reason. See the busy mind of God rejoicing at the beautiful work of his machinery, cutting and designing forms for fowls of the air and fish of the sea. Thus we are admonished to allow no opportunity to pass by of remembering the great injunction, "Despise not the day of small things." I am – I was without beginning of days or end of time – eternally the same law. My greatest stones from foundation to dome are atoms in all superstructures wherein life prevails. Animals, fish, and fowls, angels and worlds, are atoms of which you are composed. They are the associated millions which complete worlds of the greatest magnitude, without which the eye that beholdeth the same could not behold their beauties. Therefore be kind in thought to the atoms of life...*

**—A. T. Still,**
***Autobiography of A. T. Still*, Chapter XVI, page 253**

**all worlds**
**-PRESS-**

**allworldspress.com**